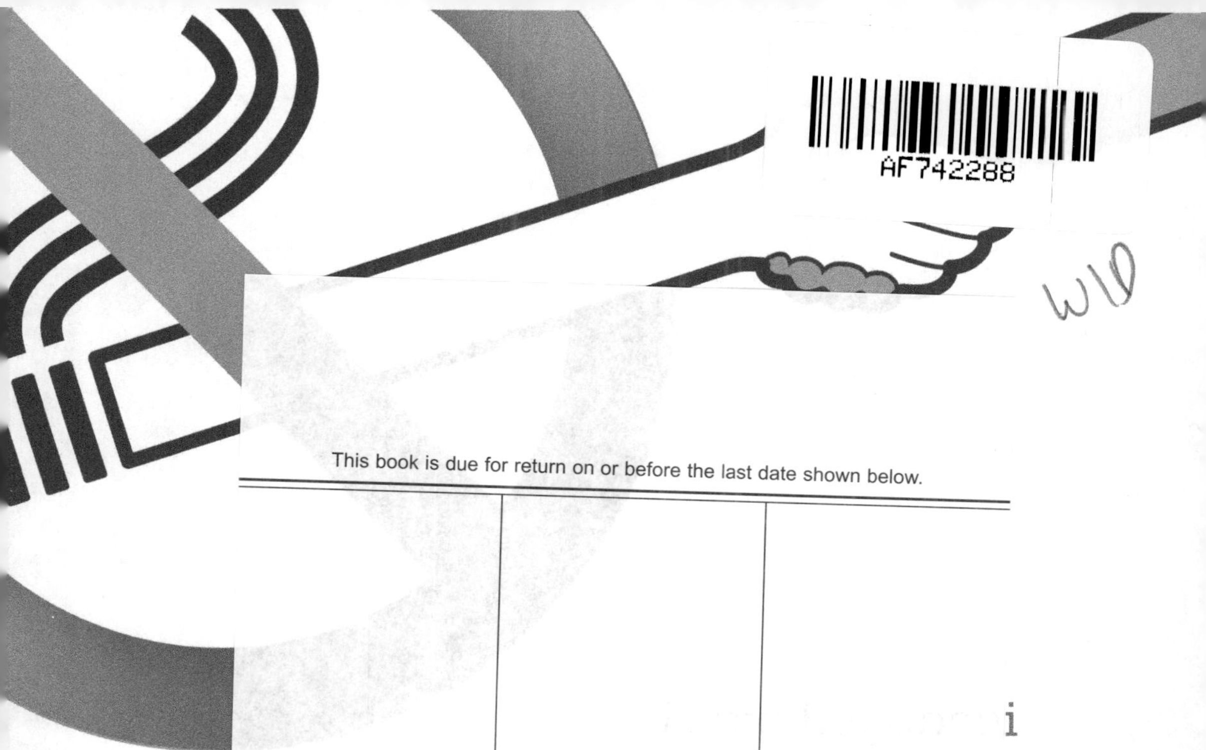

i

t

s

easy

© SE*Ed* srl
Via Magenta, 35 – 10128 Torino (Italy)
Tel. +39.011.566.02.58
www.edizioniseed.it
info@edizioniseed.it

First edition
October 2012

Title of the original Italian edition:
"Aiutare a smettere di fumare? È più facile di quanto pensi", SE*Ed*, 2012

ISBN 978-88-9741-933-4

To **Paolo Mezzelani**,

who played an important role in my life and in medicine.
Without him I would not have even thought about working on addictions;
without his advice I would have become a radiologist

Table of Contents

Preface

I often ask smokers who are facing the process of quitting smoking what the main obstacle is, the situation that—according to them—holds the greatest risks to make them miss their target. Unequivocally the answer is: the fear of not succeeding. Later, much later, comes the problem of the withdrawal syndrome, the fear of gaining weight, and other "phantoms." The situation is no different for health professionals, especially doctors. They too often stop because of their fear of failure, or get discouraged, thinking they might not have the skills to help people quit smoking. These two difficulties are also frequently reported as "lack of time." The result, unfortunately, is that the "leading cause of preventable death in the developed countries" (according to the World Health Organization [WHO]) is often left untreated. At best, the result is a referral to the closest Tobacco Treatment Center, or the paternalistic prescription: "You must stop smoking." In fact, the treatment of smoking is within the reach of health professionals, if they have a basic knowledge about drugs of proven efficacy, the correct mode of communication with the patient, and some skill of motivational interviewing. The merit of this work by Fabio Lugoboni is to make everything easily accessible and clear. Since the resources of the Health Service are increasingly limited and the tasks assigned to the GP (general practitioner) are increasingly growing, it is crucial to achieve results in outpatient settings. Treating a person with dependence on tobacco is one of the most beneficial actions in terms of cost/benefit, reduced relapse, more long-lasting health, and convenience (in terms of time spent), especially when compared with the treatment of other chronic and disabling conditions. This practical guide comes from the clinical expertise of a leading Italian expert on dependencies. Although the style uses many personal dialogues, this book is not simply a "common sense" approach, but is based on the most rigorous scientific evidence, and will be able to satisfy the need for updates of colleagues in the complex field of smoking.

Biagio Tinghino
President of the Italian Society of Tobaccology

Introduction

How This Book Was Conceived

I think it is worth briefly describing how an idea is born: it may satisfy the readers' curiosity, and I believe it is part of an author's duty toward his readers.

I am a doctor, and curing smoking addiction has been one of my main interests for many years.

I have read Allen Carr's bestseller "The Easyway to Stop Smoking"; a great number of smokers have also done so, giving overall a positive judgment of the points it puts forward. A considerable percentage of these people were also successful in giving up smoking. Doctors, if we exclude those who read it for personal reasons, have basically ignored the book, even those doctors who actively and frequently deal with smokers.

I read Carr's book four years ago while I was in a remote mountain village in Tajikistan on a humanitarian project. I remember that, as soon as I had finished the book, with a resolution unusual for me, I opened my travel notebook and started jotting down the first lines of a future book which I envisaged as having the polemic title "Giving Up Smoking Is Not at All Easy!" I wanted to make clear the excessively simple way in which Carr invited his readers to give up smoking, without following any form of treatment, after demolishing the myths connected to smoking one by one. Years of work encouraged me to do so, even if the clear, effective language and the initiatory fascination the author exerted on his readers could not be easily forgotten. I gave up smoking years ago but Carr had not caught my attention for this, rather what had attracted my interest were the trenchant visions he put forward, with his definitely remarkable ability to use a global language, considering the worldwide success of the book.

Carr's shamanistic-like approach to his reader-smoker (of the kind "Do **exactly** as I tell you and you will **certainly** succeed") tends to make those who deal with tobacco addiction turn their noses up, forgetting that such an approach has been for thousands of years the only medicine, and that any new drug has to be double-blind tested in an attempt to weigh its effect versus that of a placebo, a very expensive procedure which often yields limited differences.

That idea of a book, born as a reaction to the scientific limitations of what Carr had written, remained confined in my Tajikistan notes, developing little by little into this book aimed not at smokers but at those trying to treat them, attempting to recuperate Carr's style, rather than demonizing it.

Everything said about Carr's book—that it is irritating in its certainties, apodictic, unscientific at times—may be true, except that it is boring or unclear. Unfortunately, most of the books and articles written in order to convince reluctant general practitioners (as for hospital doctors, I would characterize them as openly resistant) to treat their patients for smoking have given me the impression of being generally boring, correctly following the rigid guidelines put forward in the scientific literature, but at the same time heavy-going, not very trenchant, and difficult to memorize. Thus the gap between the need for help, not always expressed, of the enormous number of smokers, and the offers of support often badly formulated by their doctors, remains wide.

Who This Book is for

I have been dealing with smoking addiction for 15 years and have been lecturing at university on this subject for 12. Even if I am responsible for one of the most attended anti-smoking centers in Italy, I am firmly convinced that the ideal "tobaccologist" is the smoker's doctor, his GP if he is relatively healthy, the hospital doctor (cardiologist, pneumologist, etc.) if his conditions are poor.

This conviction derives from the fact that treating a patient with a good motivation to give up smoking is relatively easy for everybody (even if things become more difficult the greater the tobacco addiction); and this has meant that a wide variety of doctors, psychotherapists, behavioral therapists, herbalists, not to mention pranotherapists and those selling many different and highly imaginative remedies have become famous. Unfortunately, motivated smokers are few and far between: most tobacco addicts have an ambivalent attitude which can be summed up as "Sooner or later I shall give up smoking, but not today." This ambiguity, typical of all forms of addiction, is often misunderstood by doctors who clearly see the priority of the damage but little understand the complexity of addiction. This rubber curtain, rich in contorted thoughts about smoking-induced damage, may be penetrated if the patient is emotionally involved by a relevant event: this could be an illness, or a sudden worsening of a condition, or a dangerous situation that has been avoided. Thus no one other than a cardiologist who is treating a smoker with a heart attack, to give an example, will have a greater influence in overcoming this ambivalence and helping the patient attain **permanent** abstinence.

Learning to treat smoking addiction is not difficult. The drugs on offer are limited in number, quite easy to use, and safe. The attitude one should have toward smokers can be learnt quite quickly and improves remarkably with time. It is an activity that yields great satisfaction to those who treat them, because smokers do not forget those who helped them to give up smoking. So what is necessary? Interest, as with anything, and time. Yes, **time**!

I have underlined this point not because it is a fundamental component—in actual fact, if well used, the time necessary for this kind of activity is very limited—but because the question: "How much of my time will all this take up?" will probably be the first one all readers, especially doctors, will ask themselves. I shall go back to this point later on, but I did want to reassure my readers.

As regards interest, I hope this book may be taken into consideration by health workers, even if not medical graduates—and by this I mean chemists, nurses, physiotherapists, behavioral therapists, psychotherapists, and all those who come in contact with the difficult condition of a smoker who wishes to give up smoking but is not able to. This is because most of the drugs can be bought over the counter, thus putting, for example, a behavioral therapist on the same strategic level as a doctor.

I have also thought about all those families who feel powerless and can only watch the apparently voluntary self-destruction of the smoker—understanding that there exists a logic in the situation, and that each smoker has a chance, and that learning which is the best way to use this chance, even if not necessarily in the first encounter, is not something to be neglected.

Methodological Introduction

Books dealing with smoking addiction usually begin with a chapter on smoke-induced damages and on how much good giving up does. The author then moves on to explain the phenomenon of nicotine addiction, the social costs of smoking, and so on. I consider this approach, which I still use with my students, rather boring if aimed at therapists, even if these subjects cannot be disregarded. I therefore decided to deal with them in the second part of this book ("The Theory"), where those particularly interested in knowing more about it can easily get information from scientific data put forward by true experts in the field. The second part also contains a detailed in-depth analysis of the motivational process, with a description of the skills useful in keeping the patients' resistance and ambivalence low; these points will also be summarized as much as possible in the main part of the book.

All that is necessary to start treating smokers will be found in the first part of the book ("The Practice").

The question of treatment is therefore approached immediately. I imagined (and this was not at all difficult since I often find myself in exactly this situation) my reader sitting next to me during and after the visit we carry out in our smoke surgery. Thus, I shall imagine you, reader, to be a doctor wishing to learn how to treat smoking addiction from scratch. Don't be offended if you aren't doctors; after all, the question is basically the same no matter who is involved. Consider that there are very few medical universities that devote even a few hours to explaining tobacco addiction, and fewer still that teach how to treat it.

I shall always try to be simple and clear, practical without forgetting the guidelines for scientific correctness. If I manage to, I would like to be an Allen Carr, explaining the guidelines set down by Michael Fiore, the author of the American guidelines for giving up smoking.

I will try to always support statements with references, even if I have chosen not to interrupt the flow of the text with reference numbers, a thing which causes some mental resistance in the researcher. After all, I am, and am proud of being, first of all a clinician. In the second part, where I shall be using a more academic tone with my colleagues, references will document every statement requiring them, and a specific list will appear at the end of each chapter.

I have used many tables, since the material is very rich and is suited to summarize the basic concepts. In addition, holding lectures on smoking is part of my job.

Part I

THE PRACTICE

Health Workers and Smoking

Fabio Lugoboni [1]

[1] Department of Internal Medicine, Medical Unit for Addictive Disorders, University of Verona, Policlinico GB Rossi, Verona, Italy

The most dangerous drug from a social point of view? Alcohol. The most damaging for the single person? Heroin. But the most lethal substance, in that it contributes to the highest number of deaths? Undoubtedly tobacco smoking, responsible in the world for one death every 10 seconds. Every smoker, if he doesn't quit, will have 14 years of his life taken away from him.

"Indeed it is difficult to identify any other condition that presents such a mix of lethality, prevalence and neglect despite effective and readily available interventions." These words are the first lines of the American guidelines for the treatment of smoking addiction.

In Italy the percentage of doctors who smoke varies: in a study carried out a few years ago on 938 pneumologists, 26.5% were smokers. Male doctors smoke as much as other graduates, following the trend described for the level of education; whereas female graduates in medicine smoke more than other graduates, as shown by the figure of 42% found in a study among female graduates in medicine in southern Italy. In other words, being a doctor does not offer any protection against smoking; on the contrary, being a doctor and a woman appears to be a risk factor.

Prevention and educational campaigns are important. One should, however, remember that in the United States, a country known for its 30-year fight against smoking, **23% of the adult population are still smokers; and also that among youngsters the percentage of smokers is above 20%**. These data once again suggest that prohibition is not a valid method to solve problems tied to addiction to psychoactive substances. It is more useful to aim at widespread information and accessibility to treatment though respecting the rights of both smokers and non-smokers.

It is time to ask you an important, but not fundamental question: Do you smoke?

The USA, which has made the fight against smoking a priority health objective, is a country where only 2% of doctors smoke, the same prevalence as found in the UK, and where no patient will ever see his doctor light a cigarette, even if he does belong to the small minority of smokers. "It would be unprofessional, like examining a patient with dirty hands. In your country more than 20% of doctors smoke, as does the remaining population, and it is a desolating daily picture to see staff smoke in hospitals." This is what Professor Michael Fiore, the greatest authority on the fight against smoking in the USA, said to my students at the University of Verona. Exactly, the university. This shows he also knows Italy well. Why is smoking disregarded as a disease in the medical degree course? After all, smoking is responsible for more than 80,000 deaths in Italy every year. The treatment of smoking addiction, which is a real disease, must become essential knowledge for all graduates, as happens for cardiovascular diseases, diabetes, etc. Even if everybody knows that cigarette smoking is bad for you, it is still classed as a "habit" or a "bad habit" and not as a disease; smoking addiction, identified by the WHO, is the main preventable cause of death. Unfortunately, Italian doctors, who do not consider giving up smoking a priority for their patients, are smokers in a percentage similar to that of the general population. It is therefore important to create, among the various people involved, a synergy for greater awareness and education, by modifying wrong beliefs and teaching good behavior practices and effective pharmacological, educational, and psychological strategies.

Briefly, coming back to what concerns us, what is fundamental is not that you do not smoke, but that, if you are a smoker, none of your patients ever see you smoke and that the working environment is totally smoke-free. Allow me to urge you, even if you smoke only a few cigarettes, in the same words Michael Fiore used with my students: "Give up smoking: it is unprofessional for a health worker." This is obviously true for all health workers.

The Smoker: A Stranger

Fabio Lugoboni [1]

[1] Department of Internal Medicine, Medical Unit for Addictive Disorders, University of Verona, Policlinico GB Rossi, Verona, Italy

Who is standing in front of us? A person with a bad habit he has difficulty losing? A person who does not care about his health? A person who likes risks? Certainly not. Smoking is not a bad habit; it is a form of addiction, and therefore a disease classified in the Diagnostic and Statistical Manual of Mental Disorders (DSM-IV) (Table I).

It is obvious that a smoker lights his first cigarette because he wants to, but it is a mistake to think that to continue smoking is a truly willful and free act. Carr puts forward a very good example of this: the action of deciding to go to the cinema is not the same as spending one's whole life in a multiscreen cinema. Smoking one's first cigarette affects certain areas in the brain in such a way as to, in an almost imperceptible manner, create conditioning and make buying a notoriously dangerous product acceptable. Imagine just for one moment picking up a yoghurt at the supermarket and seeing these words highlighted on it: "This yoghurt kills.'

Psychological addiction	Physical addiction
• There is a persistent desire or unsuccessful efforts to cut down or control substance use • A great deal of time is spent in activities necessary to obtain the substance, use the substance, or recover from its effects • Important social, occupational, or recreational activities are given up or reduced because of substance use • The substance use is continued despite knowledge of having a persistent physical or psychological problem that is likely to have been caused or exacerbated by the substance	• The user develops tolerance to the substance, as defined by either of the following: (a) a need for markedly increased amounts of the substance to achieve intoxication or the desired effect; or (b) markedly diminished effect with continued use of the same amount of the substance • The user experiences withdrawal, as manifested by either of the following: (a) the characteristic withdrawal syndrome for the substance; or (b) the same (or closely related) substance is taken to relieve or avoid withdrawal symptoms

Table I. DSM-IV criteria for psychological and physical addiction

You would undoubtedly be horrified. The mechanism will be explained in detail and in a scientifically traditional manner in the Chapter 13 by Prof. Chiamulera. What is important at this moment is to clarify some basic concepts in order to get rid of any misunderstandings or doubts. Nicotine is certainly a drug from all points of view and is difficult to give up for a variety of reasons. First of all, once inhaled, it reaches the brain very quickly (about 8-10 seconds, more quickly than an intravenous [IV] injection) and therefore complies very well with the definition that a drug is more dangerous the faster its psychoactive action. In addition to this, cigarettes give the smoker the possibility of acquiring perfect drug control much more effectively compared to other drugs. This means that the smoker, through the frequency and intensity with which he inhales, can perfectly dose the substance according to his psychophysical needs: more nicotine if he feels restless, and the nicotine will have a relaxing effect; less nicotine if he requires a stimulating action. If you think about it just for a moment, you have seen your friends who smoke (or who smoked) do exactly that: they smoke slowly and calmly when they are relaxed, but chain-smoke when they are stressed out. From a biochemical point of view, abstinence crises manifest themselves in nicotine addicts with a neurohormonal storm caused by the marked decrease of dopamine at the level of the accumbens nucleus in the mesocortical-limbic system, with a consequent intense stimulation of the prefrontal cortex, which initiates a spasmodic search for a cigarette (drug seeking behavior—think of the smoker who can't find his cigarettes and starts touching his pockets and rummaging in drawers, becoming more and more frenetic even if, for example, he is already late) accompanied by an increase in the adrenergic tone: the unpleasant feeling of being ... in danger of dying without actually being so. All this disappears immediately with the lighting of a cigarette; in other words, just what happens with a drug of abuse. This is its correct name, even if it is sold legally. The term craving describes the desire, almost always unbeatable, of taking drugs, in this case of smoking. Craving is the main manifestation of addiction. This will help you understand some of the phenomena that accompany treatment failure and relapses. Craving can be:

- **Induced by lack of nicotine**; well, quite obvious: "I haven't smoked for three days and I'm dying for a cigarette!"
- **Induced by nicotine**; less obvious: "I haven't smoked for three months and don't think about smoking often; yesterday, however, out of curiosity I lit a cigarette and today—damn!—I'm dying for another one!"
- **Induced by stimuli connected to cigarettes**: "I have successfully stopped smoking for three months but today, here in the pub with my friend John, whom I haven't seen for months (how many cigarettes we smoked together as students!), I'm dying to ask him for a fag."
- **Spontaneous**: "I haven't smoked for three months and I don't usually miss it. Today, I don't know why, but I'm dying for a cigarette!" The associated stimulus is not recognized at a rational level, as in the previous case, but remains at a subliminal level. The patient tends to feel defenseless, prey to illogical events he does not control.

It is a good idea to explain to the patient these simple phenomena which are—and you must remember this—temporary. Allen Carr, in one of the examples his readers remember most, describes addiction as a little monster a smoker has inside that pesters him, whining to be fed with smoke: "The only way you can beat it is to starve it: don't smoke and it will die!" [Carr, 2003]. In actual fact he will fall asleep, just like Sleeping Beauty in the fairy tale, and will wake up only by kissing ... a cigarette. The little monster has been asleep inside me for years and I have no intention of waking it up.

In order to become established, addiction needs a certain number of attempts, just as a fisherman must throw his line into the water several times before catching a fish. How many? Difficult to say. Studies differ on this; we are genetically different, and we live with different people. Nobody will start smoking without a smoker near him. Just to give you an idea, I could say 100 cigarettes; this is the quantity certain studies use to discriminate between smokers, ex-smokers, and nonsmokers, defined as those who have smoked less than 100 cigarettes in their life, since it is difficult to find somebody who has never smoked a cigarette in all his life. A certain number of cigarettes is important to feel an effect, ruling out any emulative aspect, we shall call **reinforcement**. The stronger the reinforcement (it helps me concentrate, it makes me less shy, it helps me remain thin, etc.), the faster addiction will set in. Smoking is not always pleasant; sometimes it can be

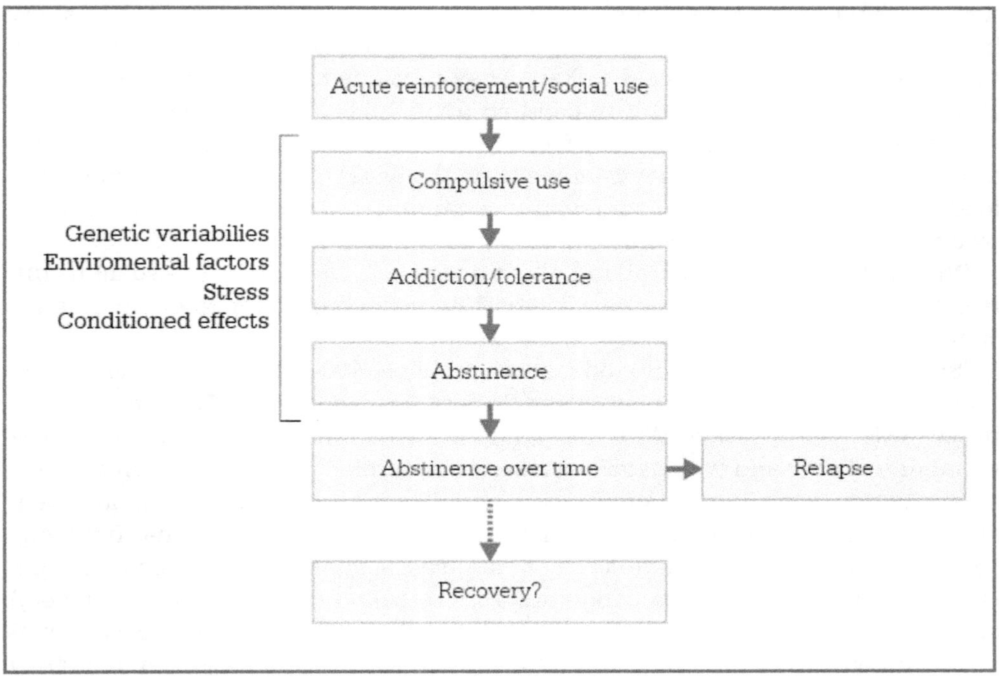

Figure 1. Genesis of addiction [Le Moal, 2007]

quite unpleasant. By continuing to smoke, the young man (because in most cases young people are involved) is able to put smoking in the right place for him, beginning with small episodes of cigarette abuse ("I don't normally smoke, but at parties I may smoke four or five cigarettes.") which start to create the phenomenon of **tolerance**. Understanding tolerance is simple and complex at the same time; all you need to know is what you already know, what everybody knows: you get used to some substances, as occurs with a glass of sweet wine, pleasant for somebody who is not a teetotaler, unpleasantly intoxicating for somebody who is. Tolerance, a creeping phenomenon if one doesn't indulge in marked abuses, makes the brain more sensitive to the gratifying effect of smoking (nicotine receptors increase, the antennae from traditional become parabolic) and, at the same time, more sensitive to the negative effects of lack of nicotine. In order to get round this second effect, one tends to smoke more regularly (Figure 1).

Addiction increases until it produces a true abstinence syndrome if one doesn't smoke. In such a situation the receptors "protest," "complain," just like baby birds who have been left by their mother in the nest without any food. And as soon as the mother returns with a little worm in her mouth, they start fighting. I will now tell you something before you start putting forward easily imaginable objections (I know a lot of smokers who are not like this, even if they have been smoking for years): about 50% of Italian smokers do not develop such a degree of addiction as to experience abstinence symptoms if they don't smoke—what the English call "going cold turkey", a very vivid way of describing the adrenergic hyperactivity deriving from abstinence. These subjects continue to smoke, even if they know how bad it is for them, under the illusion that they are not addicted because they have not experienced the "cold turkey." They continue to smoke to feel the effect of smoking and not to prevent impending abstinence. If they don't smoke, they do not feel the need to; rather they feel a latent "malfunctioning" condition, everything loses colour, even if they manage to do the usual things. In other words, the food is still passably good in our favorite restaurant, but service has become sloppy and the staff bad-tempered.

What is the point then of talking about a "smoker" when there are so many different varieties? Quite right, there is absolutely no point: from now onwards we shall always talk about "smokers" in the plural.

"Smokers come in different kinds, about 1 billion, 400 million," my friend Christian Chiamulera, past president of the Society for Research on Nicotine and Tobacco (SRNT-Europe) says. With this aphorism Christian summarizes the extreme variability of how and why people smoke. If you think of a grading varying from 1 to 10 and you apply it to different neuromodulators such as adrenalin, noradrenalin (mood, life tone, anxiety), acetylcholine (concentration, intestinal function), serotonin (mood, anxiety, regulation of impulses, sexuality), dopamine (pleasure, vigilance), vasopressin (neurovegetative function), GABAergic (sleep, anxiety) and glutamatergic systems (excitement), you will produce thousands of combinations. You will find the smoker who **mainly**, but not only, smokes to calm anxiety and the one who smokes to concentrate.

This should not, however, discourage you; after you have helped a few people to give up smoking, you will have an acceptable number of types of smokers at your disposal and be able to do a good job.

But never let appearances deceive you: "Giving up smoking is a process, not an event" (Karl Fagerström).

References

- Carr A. The Easyway to Stop Smoking. London: Penguin Books, 2004
- Le Moal M, Koob GF. Drug addiction: pathways to the disease and pathophysiological perspectives. *Eur Neuropsychopharmacol* 2007; 17: 377-93

3 Motivation

Fabio Lugoboni [1]

[1] Department of Internal Medicine, Medical Unit for Addictive Disorders, University of Verona, Policlinico GB Rossi, Verona, Italy

Blaise Pascal noted that men are more easily convinced by reasons they have discovered themselves than by those born in other people's minds. How many times have we heard somebody reporting as a great discovery things we had said many times without achieving any result? This is linked to our neurobiology: we remember and we learn preferentially what impresses us from a sensory and emotional point of view or what is necessary for our survival or to improve our condition. A friend of mine summarized a great scientific truth using everyday language: "In life you do everything for two reasons: for money or for enjoyment." The amygdala, a cerebral nucleus located in the limbic system, is responsible for mediating and integrating our learning. Unfortunately, smoking and many other drugs are remembered and learnt at this level. On the other hand, rational analysis of what seems to be right to do or has to be done sees a more direct involvement of the prefrontal cortex. The friction, the contrast between what unquestionably has to be done—"Considering your heart attack, smoking is real suicide" or "To continue to smoke with your breathing insufficiency will inevitably lead to oxygen treatment soon"—and addiction, considered as a disease entailing the **loss of the freedom/faculty to abstain**, produces a learning and behavior attitude based on denial or underestimation of the problem. I am sure you have heard many examples of this ("After all, it is certainly no less damaging than the air we breathe in town"). In other cases the ambivalence alternates rational statements with other incongruous statements—"What the doctor says is unquestionable, smoking is very bad for me, I can feel it when each cigarette I light makes me cough; but I won't be able to start the treatment he is suggesting before the summer holidays."

What may happen, however, is that certain factors with a high emotional value may unexpectedly rule out all resistance and produce total adherence to what was suggested.

This situation must be known, and sort of accepted, but you must not use it as an alibi for not doing anything. First of all you must clarify things, even with the most "denying" patients. You must be sure that the patient's resistance against giving up smoking is not due to lack of information on the risks he runs by smoking, on the advantages he would have if he gave up, or on the possibility of concrete treatment; in addition, you must have adequately investigated whether or not he has ever tried to give up smoking and what made him desist or relapse. All this to avoid becoming one of "those who explain your ideas to you without managing to make you understand" (Enzo Jannacci, an Italian songwriter).

Remember that dividing patients into "complying" and "non-complying" is too simplistic, particularly when the division into these two categories is permanent (the same is true for other personality features such as "funny," "punctual," etc.). Compliance is extremely variable in time and greatly influenced by the therapeutic relationship. I shall now briefly summarize, since they are easily learnt and memorized (and also because I imagine nobody ever spoke to you about them at university), the so-called stages of change which you may study in depth in the second part if you wish. I believe you will find them very useful not only to make your relationship with tobacco addicts easier, but also to see the doctor-patient relationship from another point of view. These stages are often represented as a wheel ("the wheel of change"), a wheel that moves with "clicks" varying greatly in duration (Figure 2).

The first stage is called **precontemplation**. In this stage the patient is defined as being unaware of his pathological condition: he doesn't really believe the objective data his doctor is supplying and, above all, has no intention of changing. The therapist often experiences the unpleasant sensation of a wall of indifference between the patient and himself. This wall throws his effort back at him in a way that is exactly the same and the opposite. Asking family members for help in

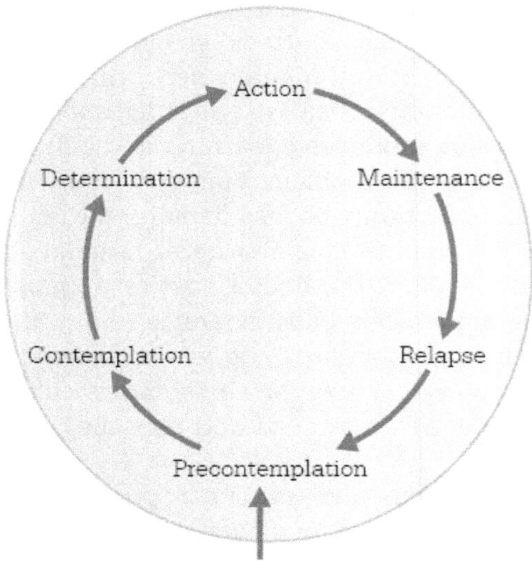

Figure 2. Prochaska's stages of change [Prochaska, 1986]

making the patient more reasonable does not yield appreciable results. One often meets patients in this stage when treating nicotine or alcohol addiction, but the same is true in the case, for example, of an exaggeratedly sedentary lifestyle or obesity.

Unfortunately, you must remember, no matter how paradoxical this stage may seem, it may last a lifetime.

The next stage, and as you will realize the term "wheel" is quite appropriate, is defined as **contemplation** and is characterized by greater awareness: the patient recognizes there are good reasons for giving up smoking, but the strong ambivalence, which is typical of this stage, tends to prevent real willingness to do so. The therapist does not experience resistance but consensus, and is warmly thanked for his efforts, but the patient doesn't even attempt to change: "Doctor, I totally agree I cannot continue to smoke. I intend to give it up after the Christmas holidays as a present for my family. For the time being, I will try to smoke a little less."

Most smokers are in this stage: they are aware of the damage caused by smoking, would like to stop, but do not feel they are ready to do so at present.

Their attitude, only apparently conciliating, may easily deceive and is annoying for the doctor who gets fed up with this continuous playing for time. But if you manage to diagnose the ambivalence of this stage you will not let yourself be led astray: it is not lack of consideration for you or arrogance; it is the patient who must become tired of making up excuses, not you, because you are the therapist and he is the patient. Be prepared, because this stage too may last a long time, in fact potentially it may never end. How many colleagues have kept on saying for years, "I want to give up smoking. I really must come and see you," every time they see me!

Continuing along the wheel of change we find the stage of **determination**, where at last the patient is determined to change. His ambiguities and his resistance appear to have dissolved just like fog does: he will accept the treatment, the therapeutic plan he has so far failed to follow. "High time too!" you might say. Quite, but you must bear in mind that, unlike the previous stages which potentially may last a long time and do not tend to evolve, determination is characterised by short duration, quantifiable approximately in terms of weeks. It is therefore vital that you notice this change in attitude, this brief moment, immediately, in order to make the beginning of the process of quitting concrete. The worst thing you can do is ... not to believe it has really arrived because you are fed up with ambivalence ("Oh, yes, it is just like many other times, big promises and then ...") This would be a mistake, and it would be a fault on your part if the patient, now seriously motivated, is not able to take advantage of your active support ("If this time you are so convinced, show me, prove your good will to me!"). The patient may be seriously motivated but fragile because of his nicotine addiction: treat him adequately and give him your support; only by doing so will you know: "The proof of the pudding is in the eating."

The stage of determination is followed by the stage of **action**: "Facts, not words!" The patient gives up smoking, overcoming difficulties and hardships. This stage does not last more than 3-6 months, not necessarily all spent in treatment, and then it moves on to the next, the stage of **maintenance**, when giving up smoking becomes a new lifestyle, often accompanied by the disbelief of the patient and of those who know him ("Incredible, Doctor, just think—I have no photo of me not smoking a cigarette!"). This stage may, hopefully, last forever.

Unfortunately, it may also evolve into the last stage of change, that rounds things up: **relapse**.

Relapse takes the patient back to a state of precontemplation or contemplation for a varying period of time, starting again from scratch or almost, forgetting the well-being he has experienced. But we shall talk about relapse later on.

Before getting to the heart of the process of quitting, I must tell you about the elements which encourage a person to change. They are basically three (Figure 3, Table II):

- **Internal fracture** ("I can't go on like this!"), the painful perception of the contradictions between the patient's present condition and what that condition should be.
- **Self-efficacy** ("I think I can change."), which is the second factor involved in change, is the confidence in one's ability to meet the objective.
- **Commitment**, the **willingness to change**, which follows the stages described above: all people are in a specific, potentially evolving, stage of change.

Try to remember this message: all three elements are necessary to change. When a smoker feels he has to change, has the feeling that he will be able to make it, and no longer postpones the decision, he is in the ideal condition for change. With a bit of support and calibrated treatment it is possible to make even severely addicted patients give up smoking. Unfortunately, however, the picture is very often incomplete. Remember also that the most important of the three factors is not

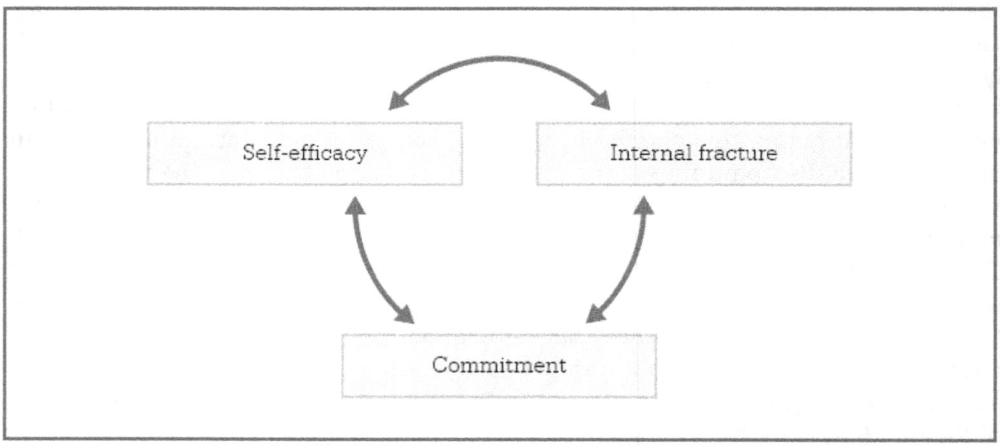

Figure 3. Schematic representation of the three elements necessary to change: self-efficacy, internal fracture, commitment (willingness to change)

Factor	Expression	Explanation
Internal fracture	"I can't go on like this"	The painful perception of the contradictions between the patient's present condition and what it should be [Festinger, 1962]
Self-efficacy	"I think I can change"	The confidence in one's ability to meet the objective in a determined period of time [Bandura, 1977]
Commitment	"I must change now"	The willingness to change and the clear perception of the problem [Prochaska, 1986]

Table II. The three elements necessary to change

the internal fracture as doctors generally think ("Considering how bad his breathing insufficiency is, you can do nothing but give up smoking!"); rather, it is self-efficacy, and your role as a therapist will be to supply, to instill, confidence, filling the gap ("I am not sure I will manage to give up smoking, it's like a mirage. But if you help me like you did with my brother I may succeed at last"). Also, the third factor, the stage of change, must not be considered an insurmountable barrier. In Canadian hospitals (the so-called Ottawa model) all smokers in hospital because of acute cardiovascular conditions are treated pharmacologically, whether they are motivated or not, so as to show them that treatment is effective and can reduce the desire to smoke (Table III).

- Systematic identification of smokers (ready/not ready/recent ex-smoker)
- Counseling
- Routine pharmacological treatment both in patients ready and those not ready to quit
- Informative material for self-help
- Follow-up: fixed contacts at 3, 14, 30, 60, 90, 120, 150, and 180 days
- Availability of phone counseling
- Link to territorial resources

Table III. Ottawa model for hospitalized patients, based on an analysis of 26 Canadian hospitals

References

- Bandura A. Self-efficacy: toward a unifying theory of behavioral change. *Psychol Rev* 1977; 84: 191-215
- Festinger L. Cognitive dissonance. *Sci Am* 1962; 207: 93-102
- Prochaska JO, Di Clemente CC. Toward a comprehensive model of change. In: Miller WR, Heather N (eds). Treating addictive behaviors: processes of change. New York, NY: Plenum Press, 1986

The Time

Fabio Lugoboni [1]

[1] Department of Internal Medicine, Medical Unit for Addictive Disorders, University of Verona, Policlinico GB Rossi, Verona, Italy

This is the first of the worries and objections that doctors bring up when they are invited to deal with tobacco addiction. When you don't know how to deal with the "job," then that mix of wavering motivations, false excuses, half-lies, but also the need for support, which is typical of smokers who wish or are "forced" to quit, is seen by doctors as extremely tiring and wasteful in terms of time; and there is always the doubt that it is all useless or that it is simply a "question of will power" on the part of the smoker. Don't feel guilty because of this: a study which involved a group of family doctors in the European Union encountered the same difficulties as described above. It also showed a widespread lack of specific university training for a problem so common and lethal as smoking addiction. These worries are normal; I feel the same when in a fit of domestic "do it yourself (DIY)" projects, I find I have pieces that do not match and the unpleasant feeling that I am wasting my time when I could be doing something much more important.

> *"Making somebody who has chosen that lifestyle give up smoking is none of my business. We all know how bad smoking is and how important it is to give up, but I don't know what to do; it's something I did not study at university. I shall do all I can to convince him to go and see a specialist even if, quite frankly, I don't think I know any."*

Factors that negatively affect general practitioner's effort to motivate his patients to quit smoking (PESCE study)

- GP thinks that smoking cessation is too time-wasting
- Necessity of specific education
- Limited ability in counselling or pharmacological therapy for cessation

Sometimes, however (and I must confess I am not very good at manual labor), I manage to succeed in my little repair job, and then I am particularly proud of what I have done. I no longer think about how long it has taken me, about the economic value of the hours spent on it; I am totally satisfied, and if my wife in passing by happens to say "Did you manage?

Clever man," even if with no particular emphasis, it may really seem a small perfect moment. You have certainly seen that smile on the face of the surgeon coming out of the operating theatre after a successful operation, which had previously been considered desperate. Helping a smoker give up smoking is indeed something more than the successful DIY job because the patient's gratefulness is usually enormous, sincere, and long-lasting. You will be surprised when years later a patient will say to you, "You made me stop smoking, Doctor. I would never have managed on my own!" You may think that this is not exactly true, that he did the hard work and that all merit quite rightly goes to him; but this will not reduce the satisfaction of having contributed to something important.

Unfortunately, you will not find the same satisfaction and gratefulness when you reduce a patient's cholesterolemia with a statin.

"Yes, okay, but how much will it cost in terms of time? I would like a more precise answer."

Not much, less than you may think. Treating smoking addiction in your patients saves time, more or less like what happens with those things we continuously postpone even if we know that sooner or later we will have to deal with them and neglecting them has a negative effect on our mind.

The patient-smoker will come to the surgery more often, will get ill more often, will weigh more on your budget compared to the nonsmoker patient, and you will have to tell him again and again about the disastrous effect of smoking (if you didn't, your conduct would be unprofessional). You will probably feel annoyingly embarrassed when he produces excuses and minimizations that are often ridiculous or when he just looks at you in painful silence.

"Okay, I have tried all this. But you are not answering my question about time. I would like to get a more precise idea."

You are quite right, and I shall try to be more precise. Your question is among the most frequent and relevant, and for this reason has been the object of a careful study. In assisted cessation an optimal cost-benefit ratio is reached with four sessions in a month. Obviously this is a rather generic statement, and later on we shall go into the details when we talk about therapeutic options, but at least you can start getting a more precise idea.

The first session will be a bit longer than the others because you will have to evaluate some important factors we shall see later on, but the follow-up sessions will be shorter, 10-15 minutes, and can be integrated with, or if necessary substituted by, even shorter phone calls.

As with all things, the more time you invest the greater the result; but since objectively the time at our disposal is limited, I would say that the time you should

> **Quit smoking: years of life gained [Doll, 2004]**
>
> - 3 years if you are 60 years old
> - 6 years if you are 50 years old
> - 9 years if you are 40 years old
> - 10 years if you are 30 years old

devote to your addicted patients who intend to quit smoking or at least want to give it a try, may basically be the following: four sessions, the first one lasting about half an hour, the other three about 10-15 minutes each, as well as short phone calls either when the patient feels the need or by appointment. Phone calls could substitute for the face-to-face sessions, but I wouldn't suggest it; it would be a makeshift solution. In total that's about 60 minutes which could allow your patient to gain many years of life, quality life with the possibility of seeing his grandchildren born or things like that, not the legendary extra week in life when it rains all week, about which Woody Allen comments ironically.

Does all this strike you as too simplistic? I shall try to be more specific. A certain number of studies have been carried out on smokers intending to quit smoking without support. Bear in mind that if you prescribe a patient an anti-smoking product and you leave him with indications such as "Let me know how things go," you are not very far from the situation of the smokers described in the studies I

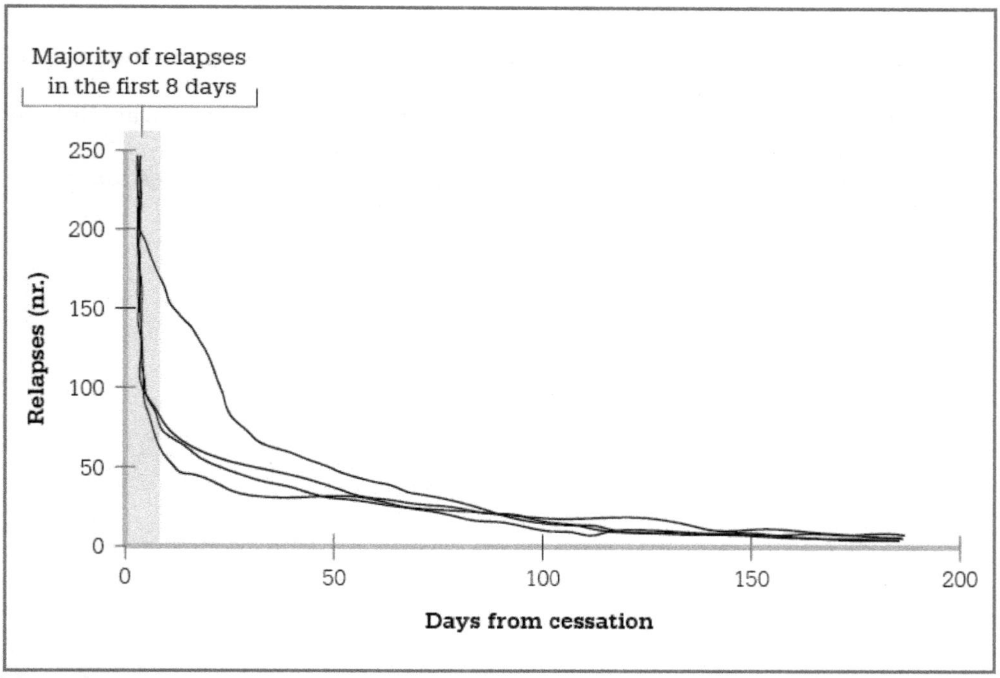

Figure 4. Quit smoking without help: data from the analysis of four studies [Hughes, 2004]

quoted. Scientific observations tell us that we shall have a relapse back to smoking in 70-80% of cases within the first week of cessation. There will be high percentages of relapse also during the second and third week; the figure will then stabilize during the fourth week. From that moment onwards a small continuous series of relapses has been observed in the abstinence survival curve, reaching an abstinence figure of 3-5% at 6 months (Figure 4).

I wish to remind you that we are talking about unsupported attempts: in supported smokers, the survival curve is similar: a higher concentration of relapses in the first 2-3 weeks, but the cessation rate is definitely higher. This is why I told you about the optimal cost-benefit ratio represented by the four sessions in the first crucial month. Obviously you will get your hand at it and this will not only allow you to gain time but also to acquire confidence. Your patients badly need to believe that it is possible to give up smoking and that, if you have managed to make other inveterate smokers quit, you must certainly know "one more than the devil!"

And this is how it will be: apart from a little essential pharmacologic ability, easy to acquire, each patient you help to quit will teach you something, until you really will have many cards to play in your hand.

References

- Doll R, Peto R, Boreham J, et al. Mortality in relation to smoking: 50 years' observations on male British doctors. *BMJ* 2004; 328: 1519
- Hughes JR, Keely J, Naud S. Shape of the relapse curve and long-term abstinence among untreated smokers. *Addiction* 2004; 99: 29-38
- PESCE. General Practitioners and the Economics of Smoking Cessation in Europe. Project Executive Summary. European Union, 2008

The Setting

Fabio Lugoboni [1]

[1] Department of Internal Medicine, Medical Unit for Addictive Disorders, University of Verona, Policlinico GB Rossi, Verona, Italy

Flexibility is everything
[Stephen Rollnick]

Before dealing with the two main topics, deciding to deal with the patient's addiction and the treatment itself, I would like to examine the problem of the setting, that is, how to deal appropriately with the patient you are going to help give up smoking. The box below lists what treatment of tobacco addiction isn't and must not be.

Treatment for tobacco addiction must not be mistaken for psychotherapy. So what is it? Simple old-fashioned treatment with medicines and words. In this field, medicines alone are not very effective, and, on the other hand, verbal support alone does not reduce the patient's suffering when in abstinence.

You'll see, you'll like it. You will find you are a bit of a shaman, in the most noble meaning of the word: an expert in medicinal herbs and in careful observation of the patient's emotions. When your words come out of your mouth, they will have an unexpected power. To achieve this (nobody is born a teacher), you will have to try and try again. I will now briefly list some recommendations that you will find are well developed in the second part and that I suggest you read. These, however, are the "rules of the game" and should be remembered. They will make your task much easier.

In helping his patients to quit smoking, the general practitioner IS NOT:

- The magic solution: "Leave it to me, I'll cure you, we have the most advanced methods!"
- The answer to the need for total care: "I'll leave you my cell phone number, you can call me any time, day or night. I'll remind you of your appointment, and if you wish, I can come to your home."
- A judge who frightens and assigns blame: "Are you aware that by continuing to smoke you have only three years of life left? Do you never think about the future of your family?"

First recommendation: **express empathy**. Empathy does not mean approval or tolerance of the patient's condition, but acceptance of the person just as he is, in the stage of change he is in. This condition of nonjudgement is the best possible compromise the doctor and the patient can produce at that moment.

Second, fundamental, recommendation: **avoid all disputes and discussions**. It is a common experience, both in life and in the medical profession, that the bitterer the discussion between two people, the less either of them is prepared to accept what had been suggested in the first place. It is as if any insistence on the part of the one who is treating paradoxically ends up reinforcing the patient's irrational defences, even increasing the initial distance between the two points of view.

Third recommendation: **get round resistance**. This derives from the observation that countering resistance head-on ends up reinforcing it, and is therefore a losing strategy. Getting round his resistance keeps the patient's defenses low and gives him the possibility of keeping his motivation as high as possible. My Tai Chi instructor says: "Resist like water," and I think this is a good example. After all, it is the same technique used in judo: to offer little resistance so as to purposely hit the points your opponent leaves unprotected and make him lose his balance. When the patient, who may be tense because he isn't smoking, tends to take it out on you or on the treatment suggested (and this happens quite frequently), let him blow off steam without interrupting him, listening to him carefully. As soon as he stops (a patient rarely speaks for more than 2-3 minutes if uninterrupted, whereas a doctor tends on average to interrupt a patient 18 seconds after he has started talking), delicately turn the question round, pointing out the positive aspects the patient has recognized or that you know are important for him:

"I am sorry the medicine made you feel sick; later on I shall tell you what to do about it. I think, however, that the words your daughter said to you yesterday evening showing consideration and encouragement are extremely important."

"It gave me great satisfaction indeed; after all I am doing all this for her."

Fourth recommendation: **work on the internal fracture**. This means to use leverage on one of the strongest spurs toward change, by acting on the patient's known contradictions (for example, the reason he suggests for giving up smoking, rather than our point of view in terms of health), not at a logical level but at an emotional one: how he feels on the one hand and how he could or should feel on the other.

"Doctor, I am afraid I won't manage. There are times when the thought of a cigarette is agony!"

"I understand you perfectly, and I assure you that it will pass. At least I no longer hear you constantly coughing; I imagine that must have been hell for you!"

"A real nightmare, I guarantee. No, I am really happy I am not smoking. With time I shall miss it less and less. Isn't that so, Doctor?"

> **The five main principles of doctor-patient communication in smoking cessation**
>
> - Express empathy
> - Avoid discussion and fights
> - Use and circumvent the patient's resistance
> - Work on internal fracture
> - Sustain self-efficacy

The last recommendation: **support self-efficacy**. This entails reminding the patient of his achievements as opposed to his difficulties, and making him feel that he can succeed. I wish to give you a simple piece of advice I hope you will remember: accompany the patient to the door when he leaves and tell him that he is doing well, that you are really pleased with how things are going. You will see how powerful an effect this simple action will have! It is quite obvious that a wavering patient benefits from frequent contact with whoever is treating him; the effectiveness of phone contacts, in the form of a proper appointment, has been shown. These contacts have produced verified advantages in giving up smoking, with very little time devoted to them.

These few lines should be read again as you get deeper into treatment. You will undoubtedly find your own way with time and practice. It will be better than others because it is your own, an expression of the way you are. Nevertheless, I suggest you read again the parts concerning the skills for the motivational interview every 3-4 months; you will find them very useful.

As basic preparation, I also suggest two techniques or, in better terms, two skills. They will not come naturally; you will have to try them out, force yourself to use them, and try them again and again, even if in actual fact they are incredibly simple. I can assure you they will become part of your professional life in other fields also.

Ask open questions. Unlike closed questions (those you can answer just yes or no or with very few words), open questions tend to stimulate dialogue.

"What makes you think the possibility of giving up smoking is inconceivable?"

rather than,

"You absolutely have to give up smoking—you do realize that, don't you?"

It may at first sight seem irrelevant, but getting used to using open questions whenever you sense resistance in your patient can give unexpected results and also bring the patient's doubts and fears to the surface, thus providing the opportunity to reassure him or to change your treatment strategy.

Listening actively consists in reformulating (in an affirmative way, without being ironical) what the patient has just said, as if it were an interesting point of view you had never considered before, even if the statement may quite frankly sound unsustainable. This puts the patient in the position of having to correct his wrong statements, without openly contradicting him, keeping his resistance low and dialogue open. In its simplest form, it means repeating what the patient has said "parrot-like," and in its most complex form, reformulating the statement as if it were preceded by "You mean to say that ..." in the affirmative form, not turning it into a question (which contains implicit disapproval). For example:

"You are saying that all smokers sooner or later go back to smoking again, so it is a waste of time to try and quit."

Almost always, as I was telling you, the patient tends to correct or reduce the impact of what he stated previously, thus opening up again a dialogue that would otherwise be already closed down:

"Well, Doctor, we all know smokers who have never gone back to smoking—you too, if I am not mistaken. I just think it is damn difficult ..."

Supporting and confirming, being able to summarize and being able to use the decisional scales are other very useful skills you can read about further on in the second part. The use of open questions and thoughtful listening are more than enough to start an honest job and achieve your first successes. What is your relational objective? That your smoker verbally commits himself to giving up smoking. Even if at first sight you think it is not much more that an illusion or a mirage ("Words and actions are wide apart!"), you have all you need at your disposal; all you have to add is a little of your time and treatment. Daryl Bem's theory of self-perception tells us that a therapist who openly and strongly takes sides in favor of change will reinforce in his patient the opposite attitude, that is, resistance to change.

Bem also suggests that "**people tend to support with their behavior the positions they defend with words.**"

The therapist, actively involved in the change, should try to encourage situations favoring change, and to avoid creating opposite situations. All this can be summarized in the expression "**to evoke self-motivating statements**"—based on the principle that, after all, we are convinced by our own words:

"Doctor, if you guarantee that the treatment you are suggesting will reduce the nervousness I have gone through every time I have tried to give up smoking ... I am prepared to give it another try."

Trust me, it works quite well. The salesmen who try to convince you either on the phone or in public demonstrations to buy something you really do not need are perfectly aware of this. These things are not taught at university, but they know them to perfection.

I have mentioned irony and would like to make myself understood more clearly. If you find yourself in the middle of a discussion with a patient you must at all costs avoid any form, even the slightest, of irony, or, even worse, of sarcasm (the difference between irony and sarcasm is, according to Hugo Pratt, an Italian comic strip author, the same as that between a sigh and a burp). Irony, if well used and in a situation of relaxed and empathic dialogue, may create complicity and give rise to laughter, which isn't in itself a bad idea.

Ah, another thing that will help you save time and make you more successful: invite your patient to find a buddy, a companion in this adventure, a shoulder on which to cry. You'll see, it won't take your smoker long to focus on it. Run through the list of possible candidates together: the ideal buddy is somebody who has already given up smoking and understands how hard it is ("If a friend of yours tells you that to give up smoking all you need is willpower, he almost certainly has never been a smoker!"), somebody who is prepared to be called on the phone when things become difficult; all in all, somebody who is there for you and happy to be there.

According to Hajek, one of the best British experts on tobacco addiction, a good buddy can result in a 30% greater chance of success.

The Actor's Suitcase

Fabio Lugoboni [1]

[1] Department of Internal Medicine, Medical Unit for Addictive Disorders, University of Verona, Policlinico GB Rossi, Verona, Italy

We have now got to the operational part of our brief training course. First of all, as in any other medical treatment (and there is no doubt that this is medical treatment), it is necessary to analyze our smoker from a diagnostic point of view.

6.1 Diagnostic Assessment

The first diagnosis that has to be made is the patient's degree of nicotine addiction. The best validated tool is the Fagerström Test for Nicotine Dependence (FTND); it is easily understood and takes only a few minutes to administer. The FTND is very specific, so you can be certain that the outcome for middle or high scores is indicative of medium or high dependence: the test photographs the situation quickly and precisely (Table IV).

On the other hand, it may lack sensitivity in cases of low levels of tobacco addiction (floor effect); therefore when the test yields very low levels (0-2), but with a nonnegligible number of cigarettes (more than 10), the test may underestimate the severity of addiction. The FTND test is self-compiling, and so in theory you could leave a certain number of copies in the waiting room. You would gain time but above all would create curiosity and reason for comparative analysis with your patients. There are two other aspects that must be investigated in the patient before giving any therapeutic indication: his motivation for change, which we have already discussed at length, and the mood the patient is in. In this case too it is not a question of a specialist's diagnosis, but of an evaluation any doctor can carry out, even if he doesn't have much time at his disposal. If I were you, I would evaluate the patient's mood even in cases where you are only in doubt. I test everybody, but realize you have a limited amount of time, so spend these 4-5 minutes in the cases where you know there may be or have been problems ("Have you ever in your life had episodes of depression, severe anxiety problems such as panic attacks, severe social anxiety, etc.?"), or if you are in doubt. It is well worth while. There are many tests available for evaluating depression. We have used Zung's SDS test because it is self-administered, very simple, and not very invasive, that is, not embarrassing. Obviously, there are many others and their significance is similar. The SDS is an old test (you can find it on the web), training time is minimal, it is used a lot by non-psychiatrists in internal medicine, and is sensitive, but not very specific. Like all tests for depression that are not specific for geriatrics, the test yields less reliable results in elderly patients. You do not have to diagnose depression, all you have to do is evaluate the likelihood that the patient will develop problematic depression during treatment.

Being diagnosed as depressed, with a precise score, generally encourages a patient to ask for help rather than step back. If a patient is depressed before he stops smoking, his condition may become worse later on, and this would make the process of giving up smoking more difficult or the probability of relapses higher. You shouldn't take what I say literally: addiction often induces depression since it makes the smoker feel totally dependent on cigarettes. In actual fact, from a methodological point of view (according to the DSM-IV), you shouldn't speak about depression if there is addiction. Psychiatrists have this clearly in mind in the case of alcoholics, but almost never in the case of tobacco addicts. Don't worry; psychia-

Questions	Answers	Points
How soon after you wake up do you smoke your first cigarette?	Within 5 minutes	3
	6-30 minutes	2
	31-60 minutes	1
	After 60 minutes	0
Do you find it difficult to refrain from smoking in places where it is forbidden?	Yes	1
	No	0
Which cigarette would you hate most to give up?	The first in the morning	1
	Any other	0
How many cigarettes per day do you smoke?	0-10	0
	11-20	1
	21-30	2
	> 31	3
Do you smoke more frequently during the first hours after awakening than during the rest of the day?	Yes	0
	No	1
Do you smoke even if you are so ill that you are in bed most of the day?	Yes	0
	No	1

Table IV. Fagerström Test for Nicotine Dependence

trists on average know very little about tobacco addiction. I do, however, strongly suggest that if you have a patient fully intending to give up smoking who is being treated for depression or who has had serious episodes of depression (even if at the moment he is in a state of well-being), you either contact his psychiatrist or send him to a specialist in tobacco addiction.

6.2 Therapeutic Options

Simple direct medical advice (minimal advice) and the use of informative material with detailed information on the dangers of smoking have been found to be relevant in making people give up smoking. But this relevance often has a very limited scope; this is why, after the quick but careful diagnosis described above, it is worthwhile considering pharmacological treatment. As you can see from Figure 5 (these are meta-analysis data from the Cochrane Library), the winning strategy is to combine drugs and support.

If it is true that pharmacological treatment can on average treble the probability of success, it is undoubtedly true that to prescribe pharmacological treatment

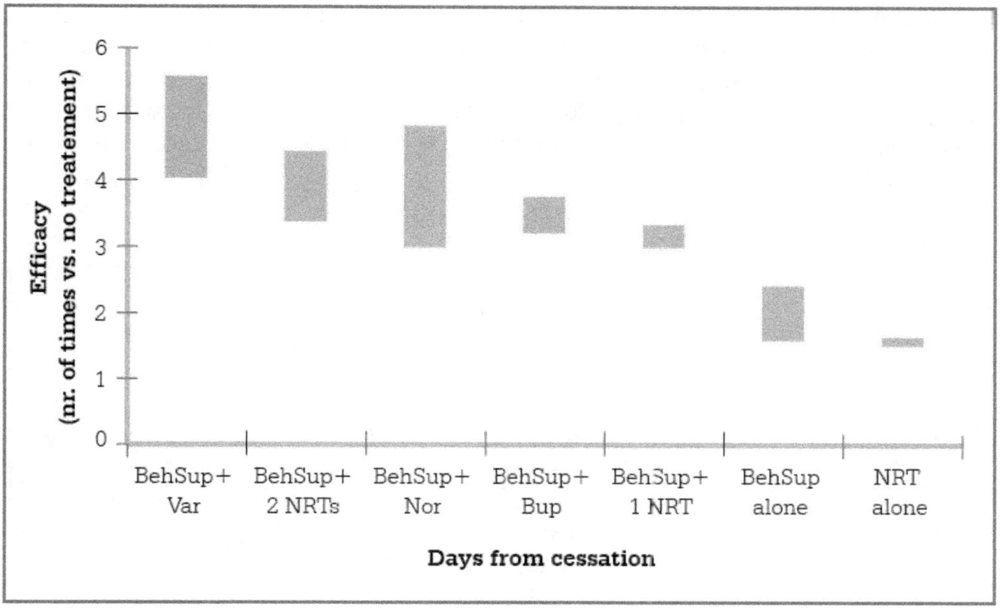

Figure 5. Current treatments: efficacy [Cahill, 2007; Silagy, 2004; Hughes, 2004]

BehSup = behavioral support; Bup = bupropion; Nor = nortriptiline;
NRT = nicotine replacement therapy; Var = varenicline

without support adds only a slight chance of success to the simple "do it yourself" approach. It is the combination of pharmacological support (aimed at reducing psychophysical distress due to abstinence) with behavioral support (aimed at keeping the patient's motivation and commitment strong) that gives the best results. Let's examine the three pharmacological treatments that have been recognized as scientifically valid for giving up smoking.

Nicotine Replacement Therapy (NRT)

Medical use of nicotine is still at the moment the most used and well-known treatment for patients who intend to give up smoking. In Italy, unlike other countries where NRT has been and is being used widely, this treatment has been little and badly applied. Perhaps because of poor information on the part of the medical profession, nicotine replacement has often been (self)administered for a few days and/or underdosed, thus making its unquestionable potentialities fruitless.

The principle on which it is based is abrupt substitution of the nicotine from cigarette smoking with nicotine introduced into the bloodstream absorbed either through the skin or through the mucosa. This, if well employed, avoids the negative effect of abstinence—let's call it the "discomfort" caused by giving up smoking, which is particularly marked, especially in the first few days after quitting, in subjects with medium or high dependence. This discomfort must not be neglected or considered of little importance ("Don't give up, in a week's time it will be gone!"), because the smoker with high dependence does actually suffer a lot and has the unpleasant feeling that time never goes by. This is why 80% of relapses in smokers who quit without any support (unfortunately the vast majority even today) occur during the first week. But now let's analyze in detail the various nicotine replacement methods (Figure 6).

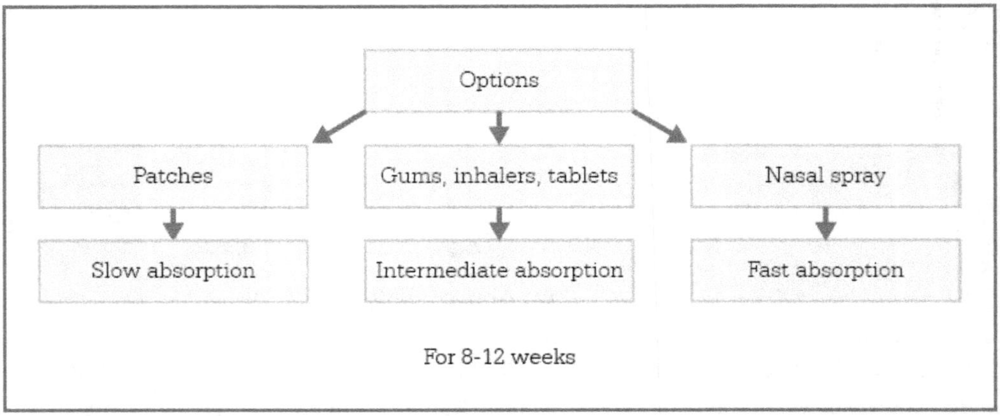

Figure 6. Nicotine replacement therapy. Modified from [Silagy, 2004]

Advantages	Disadvantages
• Discretion (you can't see them) • Well tolerated (few contraindications and side effects) • Very good action in stabilizing mood and anxiety • Remote risk of dependence	• Poor effect on appetite and on increase in weight • Insufficient release of nicotine in stressful situations or in case of marked craving • Skin rash

Table V. Nicotine patches: advantages and disadvantages

Event	Adverse events			
	Very common (≥ 1/10)	Common (1/10-1/100)	Non common (1/100-1/1000)	Rare (1/1000-1/10,000)
Disorders of the immune system	-	-	-	Urticaria, rash, itching at times generalized, angio-edema
Psychiatric disorders	-	Insomnia	Abnormal dreams	-
Disorders of the nervous system	-	Dizziness, headaches	-	-
Heart diseases	-	-	Palpitations	-
Gastrointestinal disorders	-	Nausea	Vomiting	-
Disorders of the muscular-skeletal system and of the connective tissue	-	Localized muscular pain	-	-
Systemic disorders and conditions relative to the site of application	Reactions at the site of application such as rash and itching	Reactions at the site of application such as edema and burning	-	-

Table VI. Adverse effects of nicotine patches

Four brands of **nicotine patches** are available in Italy (brands and dosages vary from different countries): Nicorette® (dosages of 15/10/5 mg/16 h), NiQuitin®, Nicopatch® e Nicotinell® (dosages of 21/14/7 mg/24 h).

Patches are applied on the skin when awakening in the morning: anywhere on the body, preferably not on hairy or irritated areas, generally starting from the first day of giving up smoking. Some patches (Nicorette®) have to be taken off at night before going to bed, whereas others (NiQuitin®, Nicopatch® e Nicotinell®) are kept on till the following morning. These different indications are due to different strategies: continuous release of nicotine at night may disturb sleep (nicotine has a stimulating effect) but avoids craving when the patient wakes up. Nicotine release is gradual and produces constant levels of nicotine in the bloodstream. It is advisable to change the place where the patch is applied every day so as to prevent skin rash. The strong point of patches is in the constant release of nicotine, but this is also the weak point of this form of treatment (Table V): the patient often tends to smoke in stressful moments when he feels a greater craving for nicotine, whereas a patient with a lower degree of dependence may be disturbed by the excessive nicotine load and suffer from nausea and palpitations. Patches and other NRT products should not be used during pregnancy, or in patients who have recently had a heart attack or who suffer from active peptic ulcer or paroxysmal tachycardia. In actual fact, these limitations are to be taken with a wide discretionary margin. In France and in the United Kingdom, these contraindications have been removed from the accompanying leaflet so as not to give misleading alibis. The message is basically this: if a patient smokes or is suffering from a severe abstinence crisis because he cannot smoke (for example, a patient in a heart unit or bedridden), the patch is clearly an advantage rather than a risk for his health (Table VI).

Most of these effects are moderate; they clear spontaneously and quickly when the patch is removed. In cases of severe or persistent skin reaction, treatment must be stopped and another type or nicotine replacement product must be used. Some symptoms, such as dizziness, headaches, and insomnia, may be a consequence of giving up smoking.

This type of treatment is the first choice when the patient has already benefited from a previous attempt, in patients who do not want to take medications, in patients with a history of major depression, and in smokers who smoke almost all the time. Patches are less useful and less tolerated in smokers with marked daily differences in the cigarettes smoked and in cases where marked weight increase is feared.

The fact that cigarette smoking when a nicotine patch is in place is absolutely not risky for the patient's health should also be pointed out.

Operative dosage: start with a 21 mg/24 hr patch, or 15 mg/16 hr in heavy or medium-heavy smokers (FTND score higher or equal to 5) and maintain this dosage, if well tolerated, for 6 weeks; then move onto the lower dosage (14 mg/24 hr or 10 mg/16 hr) for another 2 weeks; finally moving onto the final 7 mg/24 hr or 5 mg/16 hr dosage for the last 2 weeks. If in doubt continue with the higher dosage, but do not be afraid to decrease the dosage in cases of poor tolerance to the suggested dosages. Start with lower dosages (14 mg/24 hr or 10 mg/16 hr) in smokers with an FTND score lower than 5.

Advantages and disadvantages of **nicotine gums** are summarized in Table VII.

Gums, with either 2 or 4 mg of nicotine, must be chewed briefly and then kept longer in the buccal vestibule (the cavity between the lips and the dental arches)

Advantages	Disadvantages
• Faster release compared to patches and greater adaptability to different situations • Greater "orality" compared to patches • Greater control of reactive hunger, greater evidence of weight control • More personalized use • Some patients love chewing gum	• Tendency to be underused • Less tolerated than patches (local and gastroesophageal irritation, nausea, hiccups) • Not indicated in cases of teeth disorders and in patients with dentures • Not very frequent but not negligible risk of dependence • Some patients hate chewing gum

Table VII. Nicotine gums: advantages and disadvantages

for about 30 minutes so that a suitable quantity of nicotine is absorbed. The manner in which the gums are used is very important: almost all patients ignore that the gums must be chewed only until they soften a little and then kept in the vestibule. Continuous chewing increases esophageal irritation and reduces absorption. The hard palate in fact (unlike the front part of the buccal cavity) is not supplied with much blood and does not allow effective transmucosal absorption. In addition, duodenal absorption of the swallowed nicotine bolus is very slow and undergoes the "first pass" action in the liver. The 4 mg dose has been proven to be much more effective than the 2 mg dose when used as a single treatment. Gums allow the patient to vary the quantity of nicotine in the blood at different times, even if it is advisable to chew a gum at regular intervals rather than when necessary, especially considering the slowness of absorption compared to a cigarette: 10 seconds as against approximately 1000. The taste is usually described as unpleasant, although varieties with mint flavouring are available in some countries. Certain categories of workers are not allowed by their work contract to chew, for example, food dispensing staff.

As regards contraindications, the same considerations pointed out for patches are true for gums. It should be observed that for patients with coronary disorder the use of gums is safer than other NRT products which are more rapidly absorbed, since gums do not produce nicotine blood peaks.

Advantages	Disadvantages
• They are the NRT product with the fastest absorption • Generally the most appreciated by smokers and with fewer limitations • Correct use more probable than with gums (see above)	• Tendency to underuse • Not very frequent but not negligible risk of dependence

Table VIII. Nicotine tablets: advantages and disadvantages

Gums must not be given to under 18-year-olds without consulting a doctor. In adults it is advisable to start with the 2 mg gums discovering, according to the patient's needs, the best posology, i.e., the number of gums to be chewed during the day. Should the smoker tend to chew more than 15 2 mg gums a day, as in the case of heavy smokers, 4 mg gums are to be preferred. The suggested duration of treatment is 2-3 months. At the end of this period the daily dosage should be reduced. It is a good idea for the patient to have a few gums at hand should the desire for smoking suddenly return. In most smokers 10 2 mg gums a day are as a rule sufficient.

After a series of launches and withdrawals of products, 1.5 and 4 mg NiQuitin Mini® **tablets** are at the moment regularly available on the market (Table VIII. Brands and dosages vary from different countries).

Dosages depend, also in this case, on the degree of dependence and on the smoking habits of each subject. The 1.5 mg tablets are suitable for patients who smoke 20 cigarettes a day or less (FTND below 5). The 4 mg tablets are suitable for patients who smoke more than 20 cigarettes a day (FTND above or equal to 5). Tablets must be put into the mouth and allowed to dissolve, preferably under the tongue or in the vestibule. They should every now and then be moved from one side of the mouth to the other until they are completely dissolved (about 10 minutes). The tablets must not be chewed or swallowed whole. You mustn't drink or eat with a tablet in your mouth. Every time the patient feels the need to smoke, he should take 1 tablet. A sufficient quantity of tablets should be taken every day up to a maximum of 15. Continue taking tablets for up to 6 weeks to break the habit of smoking, then gradually reduce consumption. When daily consumption is 1-2 tablets, treatment must be stopped. Patients may take 1 tablet in situations when they are greatly tempted to smoke after the end of treatment. Children and adolescents: tablets may be taken by adolescents (between 12 and 17 years of age) only under medical supervision.

In Italy, **nicotine powder inhalers** are only available in the brand Nicorette Inhaler®. Inhalers are mouthpieces releasing a small quantity of nicotine powder that is predominantly absorbed in the buccal cavity. The patient must inhale to feel some benefit, but it is best to suck the inhaler rather than inhale should an irritation or cough appear (Table IX). Inhalers may be useful in patients who are strongly dependent on the gestures involved in smoking.

Advantages	Disadvantages
• Gestural component appreciated by many smokers • Fewer side effects compared to gums	• Often incorrectly used, instructions not always easily understood (cartridges not changed frequently enough, deep inhalation) • Higher risk of dependence compared to other NRTs

Table IX. Nicotine powder inhalers: advantages and disadvantages

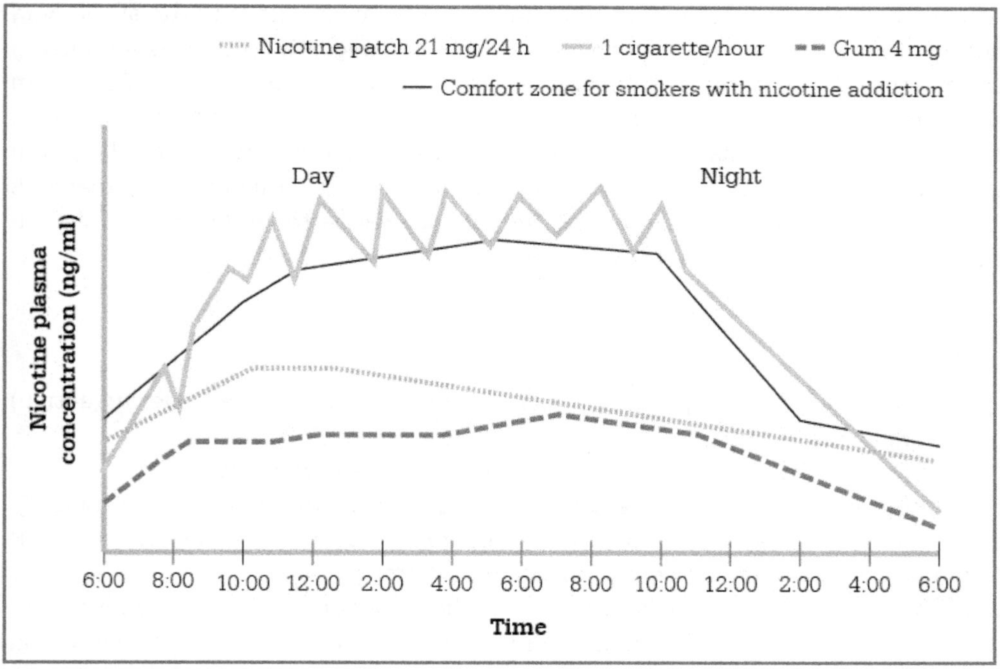

Figure 7. Nicotine plasma concentration during the first 24 hours [Bader, 2009]

The risk of developing NRT dependence, though low, should be kept in mind. It occurs more often when inhalers, gums, or tablets are used, much less frequently with patches, which are effectively employed to treat gum dependence.

The recommended dosage for adults is no less than six units a day and no more than 12 units a day. The maximum dosage is reached 20 minutes after use (continuing to inhale). Dosage is personal and depends on the need the patient has to reduce abstinence symptoms associated with giving up smoking. The suggested duration of treatment is 2-3 months. At the end of this period the daily dosage should be gradually reduced over the next few weeks (Figure 7).

Combined NRT Treatment

The association of 2 NRT products has optimized the smoker's well-being in the first, crucial weeks of the abstinence phase. The fixity of the nicotine levels in the blood supplied by patches, on the one hand, and the moderate but slow peaks given by the products to be taken when needed, on the other, complement one another in an excellent manner when they are associated.

If in the light-moderate smoker (FTND < 5) one NRT product may be enough, it is advisable to associate patches with another NRT to be taken when needed in heavy smokers. Thus the patient will have positively experienced the stabilizing action of patches but will have the possibility of integrating them by increasing his nicotine intake (tablets, gums, inhalers and sprays) when he is in difficulty. In this case the nicotine peaks will be reached faster and be more effective because of the presence of a basal level of nicotine in the blood guaranteed by the patch and, consequently, the area of "nicotine wellness" will be more easily reached. Combined NRT treatment allows tailoring of dosages better and increases the patient's responsibility, but also increases costs considerably.

Bupropion

Bupropion is an antidepressant drug (with a dopaminergic-adrenergic action) authorized in different formulations:

- bupropion SR (sustained-release): 150 mg tablets (Zyban®, Zybane®);
- bupropion XR (extended-release): 150-300 mg tablets (Wellbutrin®, Elontril®).

FDA indications are: major depressive disorder, seasonal affective disorder (XR formulation), and smoking cessation (SR formulation).

It is the same drug, the only difference is the speed of release, slower for bupropion-XR (B-XR) which is administered in a single morning dose, unlike bupropion SR (B-SR) which is taken twice a day.

It is to be noted that B-SR has been marketed all over the world as an anti-smoking drug simply by pharmacokinetically slowing down in the immediate-release bupropion the release of the compound into the bloodstream in order to increase its safety and reduce its side effects. All the studies on smoking have been carried out with the B-SR compound.

Advantages	Disadvantages
• Anti-craving action competitive with nicotine • Antidepressant action (useful in patients with an under-threshold or past depressive syndrome) • Anorectic action • Can be associated to NRT treatment	• The anti-craving effect varies greatly from one patient to another (from excellent to almost nonexistent) • Side effects not to be disregarded (nausea, tachycardia, sweating, insomnia, hypertension) • Not suitable for patients who have suffered from convulsions or who are suffering from conditions at risk for convulsions or who are taking medication that can favor such a condition • Of the front-line drugs it is the one hardest to manage

Table X. Bupropion: advantages and disadvantages

This drug is undoubtedly effective in the case of frequent contacts, even by phone, or visits to the surgery, but it is not suitable for self-management on the patient's part, both because of its side effects (e.g., hypertension) and because of the patient's need for support while he is giving up smoking (Table X). In fact, unlike NRT products, B-SR is taken for the first 8-10 days without suspending smoking, in order to adequately titrate the drug, one tablet a day for the first 6 days, then two tablets a day, at 8-12 hours intervals. There would be no sense in encouraging the patient to give up without adequate support.

The patient may at times not feel the antagonist effect of B-SR on nicotine (very variable) accurately. Because of this, it is very important to investigate, during the induction phase, not only the number of cigarettes smoked but also the depth of inhalation and whether the cigarette is smoked to the very end, remembering that the first half of a cigarette releases only ¼ of the nicotine available whereas the remaining ¾ are concentrated in the second half. In cases where the response is weak, another type of treatment, such as an NRT treatment, may be indicated. This appears to improve the outcome (controversial data). Treatment with bupropion should be continued for 8 weeks. There are not, in our experience, risks of abuse, not even in the rare cases when treatment was continued longer. The drug is rather expensive.

Operative posology: start with one tablet of B-SR in the morning, preferably on a full stomach, for 6 days, and then move on to two tablets (the second tablet should be taken preferably after 8-9 hours rather than 12, in order to limit the risk of insomnia), allowing the patient to smoke freely. Smoking should be stopped between the eighth and the twelfth day from the beginning of treatment. The exact day for cessation should be agreed upon between doctor and patient. Treatment must be continued for 8 weeks, but can be prolonged for up to 6 months (Figure 8).

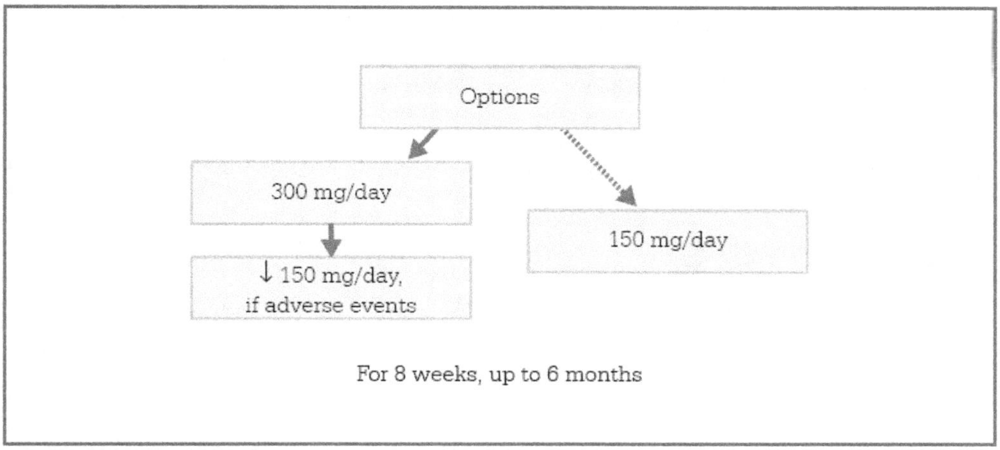

Figure 8. Bupropion (Zyban®, Zybane®) [Hughes, 2004]

Varenicline

This is the latest of the front-line drugs and at the moment the most used in specialist centers. Its commercial name is Champix® in UK and Europe and Chantix® in the USA and it is available in two packages: a starting-pack with 0.5-1 mg tablets and a 1 mg continuation pack (maintenance dose 2 mg a day).

Varenicline has, in a certain way, revolutionized the approach to smokers in specialist settings. Its strong anti-craving action, together with its powerful anti-abstinence effect, the possibility of reaching cessation of smoking gradually, accompanied by an antagonist action on the perception of smoked nicotine, has quickly made it a very popular drug among patients in anti-smoking centres. Patients often specifically ask for this drug, having heard about it by "word of mouth," very common among smokers. All this is undoubtedly true, but I feel I have to point out that prescribing this drug without adequately supporting the smoker would lead to bitter disappointment.

Operative posology: begin with the starting-pack, telling the patient to take one 0.5 mg tablet in the morning, on a full stomach, for 3 days. Increase the dose to one 0.5 mg tablet twice a day (at breakfast and dinner) for another 5 days, moving on to the maintenance 1 mg dose twice a day (at breakfast and dinner) to be

Advantages	Disadvantages
• It has been proven to be the drug with the strongest anti-craving and anti-abstinence effect available today • It is a drug with a partial agonist action on nicotine receptors, which has been specifically developed for giving up smoking; it is not an antidepressant • It is basically free from contraindications (only pregnancy and young age) • It is basically free from pharmacological interactions • It is extremely easy to use and carries only few and limited side effects • Complete cessation of smoking is reached gradually • It has been devised for a relatively long treatment course (on the whole 12 weeks), reducing the time the doctor must devote to support, without leaving the patient without support • Has been, generally, judged very positively by patients	• It is a drug and therefore must be "explained" to the patient • It is not suitable for association with other front-line drugs • It is not a first choice for smokers with major depression • Quite expensive, but the expense can be spread out, a point that is generally well accepted by patients, who do not have to buy the whole treatment course at the beginning

Table XI. Varenicline: advantages and disadvantages

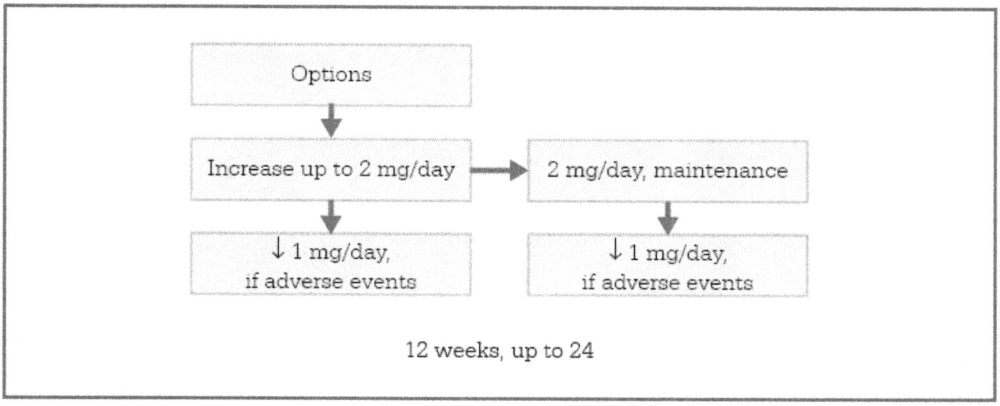

Figure 9. Treatment scheme with varenicline (Champix®, Chantix®) [Cahill, 2007]

continued up to the twelfth week, a time that can be prolonged (though this is not often necessary) up to 24 weeks. Cessation of smoking is usually agreed upon around the tenth-twelfth day. The packages (which cover 14 days' treatment, both in the case of the starting-pack and the continuation pack) are clear and the instructions easily understandable.

Of the very slight possible side effects, nausea is the most frequent and can be annoying. This is linked to the speed of absorption of the drug and not to a gastro-damaging action, therefore nausea is more similar to pregnancy nausea rather than to nausea caused by gastritis. When it occurs, it can be solved by telling the patient to eat a little more at breakfast or by dividing the doses: half a tablet at the three main meals, up to half a tablet twice a day. This strategy is usually more than enough to obtain a good pharmacological effect and good tolerance (Figure 9).

References

- Bader P, McDonald P, Selby P. An algorithm for tailoring pharmacotherapy for smoking cessation: results from a Delphi panel of international expert. *Tobacco Control* 2009; 18: 34-42
- Cahill K, Stead LF, Lancaster T. Nicotine receptor partial agonists for smoking cessation. *Cochrane Database Syst Rev* 2007; (1): CD006103
- Hughes J, Stead L, Lancaster T. Antidepressants for smoking cessation. *Cochrane Database Syst Rev* 2004; (4): CD000031
- Silagy C, Lancaster T, Stead L, et al. Nicotine replacement therapy for smoking cessation. *Cochrane Database Syst Rev* 2004; (3): CD000146

Behind the Desk, Back to Work

Fabio Lugoboni [1]

[1] Department of Internal Medicine, Medical Unit for Addictive Disorders, University of Verona, Policlinico GB Rossi, Verona, Italy

Okay, ready to start. Now we have to imagine a patient standing here in front of us. I suggest you start with patients who are motivated, patients you know, patients on which you have a certain influence and whom you particularly care for. This will allow you to become familiar with the pharmacological treatments and with the setting. After treating about 30 patients of this kind, you can start with more ambivalent and complex smokers. When you feel completely at ease with smokers (that is to say when you become good at it) you can also deal with the difficult smokers, those who also have a psychological condition. Let's not fix any limits. Let's imagine the following conversations where I have written down only the therapist's words, that is yours, leaving you to imagine the patient's answers.

7.1 Case A

Routine visit to a general practitioner

"Dear Mr. Smith, you suffer from arterial hypertension and you will have to take medication. Do you smoke?"

"So, 15 cigarettes a day. It is very important you stop smoking altogether, as soon as possible. This will improve the effect of the medication and greatly reduce the suffering of your cardiocirculatory system. I am prepared to help you."

"You do well to seek help. Specific treatment will help you by greatly reducing your desire to smoke and minimizing the effects of abstinence from smoking. Shall we set up an appointment? Um, next month strikes me as being too far away. Shall we make it next week? Right, it will take 20 minutes, no longer. Fill in this simple test at home. It's a Fagerström test and will quantify

precisely your degree of dependence. Bring it on Tuesday and we can evaluate it together. Talk about it with your wife and children. No, don't be afraid of losing face if you don't manage to give up smoking. Talking about it with the people closest to you will help and will stimulate you, not hamper you. Nobody will force you to do anything: we will simply help you to accomplish something that is not easy, but is essential. See you on Tuesday."

First visit

- *"Right, so here we are. So this is the test you filled in. Let's see ... Your score is 6. Um, even if you don't smoke a lot of cigarettes, your urge to smoke is quite high. Don't worry, it's only a question of finding the right kind of treatment."*
- *"Have you ever given up smoking? Did you take anything in 2005 when you stopped smoking for a week? Nothing, you took nothing. You say it was really difficult and you were very short-tempered. Then you lit a cigarette at a time when you were particularly short-tempered and you started smoking again."*
- *"I feel I can reassure you: I think things will be different this time if we give it a try together."*
- *"What is your main reason for wanting to give up smoking? Don't say something just to please me, as your doctor. Feel free to answer truthfully. Ah, your daughters: you would feel less pestered by your two daughters. I understand, it is not pleasant to be constantly reproached, so much that you end up by being ashamed of smoking."*

The patient's true motivation is memorized or noted down: it will be the guiding motif all through treatment, the spur which will allow us to stimulate the patient at difficult times, when his motivation weakens, rather than using medical reasons (hypertension, for example) which are not so strong when they are not also the patient's priority.

- *"Have you had episodes of severe depression during your life? Have you had episodes of marked anxiety such as panic attacks, social anxiety, etc.? No? Good. I suggest you take this medication. You can start taking it tomorrow and keep on smoking. No, this is not a contradiction, the medication will slowly reduce your desire for smoking. It may change the taste of cigarettes, so it will be easier to give up. But we'll discuss all this next time, in 10 days' time; it will only take 10-12 minutes. Don't worry, it is not a psychotropic drug. Its action is on the place where nicotine has its effects. The cost?*

What you spend on cigarettes ... But it can be deducted from your tax return as a medical expense. See you next time. Ring me if you feel the need. Goodbye."

As you have probably worked out, I suggested treatment with varenicline. Its manageability and its effectiveness make it the first choice in surgery settings. Needless to say, I would like you to be able to use all the different anti-smoking treatments after a short period of time, but it is better to use more effective and safer tools to start with.

First checkup

"So, Mr. Smith, how did things go? Did you have any problems in tolerating the medication? Only three cigarettes yesterday! Very good. Now we have to decide on the day when you will stop smoking. In order to stop, one has to ... stop. I'd say, Christmas isn't very far away, 40 days. No, three cigarettes a day are not particularly harmful, but they do not do you any good, that's for certain. The point is that in order not to want to smoke, you must not smoke. One cigarette leads to another, as I'm sure you understand."

"Do I have to decide? I suggest you stop smoking next Monday; it will be the beginning of a new week and of a new life. Goodness knows how happy your daughters will be."

"Right. This is what I would do: continue taking the medication and smoke freely until Sunday evening. Before going to bed get rid of all the remaining cigarettes. You must get up on Monday morning without having any at hand. No, don't keep any as a memento, not even as a challenge. They would be a dangerous stimulus; and anyway, whoever would fill the fridge with cakes before starting a diet? Ok, so that's agreed. Another thing: find somebody close to you who has stopped smoking, and who is prepared to answer the phone or talk to you, should you need to when you stop smoking. Your brother? Does he keep getting on at you about smoking? Many ex-smokers are like that and it's not nice for somebody who smokes, but this time he could give concrete support if you need it, you'll see. The presence of a buddy (that is a shoulder to cry on) has been proven to improve the chances of being successful in giving up smoking by 30%. We must have your brother on our side, get him involved."

"Right, see you the following Monday; yes, seven days after you have stopped. No, it's not too soon. I want to see if everything is going well; 10 minutes will be enough. You can also ring me if you need to. See you soon, and good luck."

Second checkup

"Well, how did it go? You can't believe you've stopped, can you? This is how it usually works out. Now it's important not to light a cigarette at pleasant times. I suggest you don't drink alcohol for a few days—let's say a couple of weeks; this will make you more alert when you are in the company of other people. You see, even a single glass of wine can make you be off your guard. You wouldn't want to sign a contract for a job with a difficult client after having had a drink, would you? As for coffee, that's not a problem; you can drink as much as you like, unless you feel the combination is irresistible. You'll see that when you stop smoking, you will automatically drink less coffee. Ah, you've already noticed it; good. Anything else? Good. Okay. See you in 10 days' time then and ... you've done really well!!"

Playing on self-effectiveness, increasing the patient's feeling that he will manage, is one of our tasks in the first stages of treatment. A bit at a time we'll tend to direct attention to the relevance of cessation, to keep the value of what has been achieved high, and to increase motivation.

Third checkup

"Everything all right? You had a bit of nausea and aren't sleeping very well? Well, you stopped smoking only 17 days ago and you were saying that you've been sleeping normally these last couple of days. Yes, these are usually temporary problems. The nausea could be a consequence of the medication. Always take it on a full stomach, especially in the morning. Yes, nothing particular, just a slightly bigger breakfast, not just a cup of coffee. If it doesn't disappear, we can reduce the dose, but I'd rather wait a few days more. Your brother can't believe it? And what about your daughters, what do they say? I understand. It's a great satisfaction for a father."

"You wonder why you feel so little like smoking? Well, I'd say for 2 reasons: first, you are taking specific medication; second, because you aren't smoking. Your brain is ... healing, but you'd get used to smoking again if you tried lighting a cigarette. Better to 'let sleeping dogs lie.' I'd say we could meet in 2 weeks' time—yes, always for 10 minutes. Um, better in person than on the phone. Maybe we can talk on the phone after that. Let's do things the right way. Everything is going so well!"

The patient who feels well may now tend to underestimate his commitment. The risk of a relapse is still high for the whole of the first month, so better to see him personally, leaving telephone support for later on, if possible.

Fourth checkup

"So this is the fourth time you've come since we started. Everything's all right, I think. The nausea is getting better and you are sleeping like a log—good. Ah, you've put on two kilos. I'll tell you something: it's quite normal; but usually the price to pay is no more than 2-3 kilos. You'll lose them in 2-3 months, but do try not to put on any more. Don't be discouraged, follow these dietary indications, and do a little more exercise. Do you know how many cigarettes you haven't smoked in this last period? 400! Surprised, aren't you? I know. One never thinks about it in these terms, but this is the truth. Tell your daughters and your wife. What a success! And you say you aren't as short of breath as you used to be—not bad. Your blood pressure has also improved. I think we can wait a bit longer before starting on medication for that, but I can't promise it won't be necessary. We'll see. No, you don't need to worry about when we stop the anti-smoking medication: it will be like taking the plaster off when the fracture has mended. I think we can speak on the phone in 20 days' time, or by mail, what do you think?"

As you can see, the content of these exchanges becomes more and more similar to your daily exchanges with patients in the surgery, and I have less and less advice to give you. Oh, but I do have another small piece of advice: keep your patient hooked, if you can, even if only with short phone calls. You should contact him every 15-20 days. These contacts are like the slight, but necessary, adjustments a helmsman applies to the helm. See your patient when he stops taking the medication; it will help to make him understand what you have achieved together, and show him that you will be at hand in case of relapse. Keep on asking him if he is smoking each time you see him.

Shall we have a look at another patient together? As before, I shall write down only the questions, leaving the reader to guess the answers.

7.2 Case B

Routine visit to a general practitioner

"Good morning, Mrs. Smith. I am a bit worried about the results of your blood tests. You suffer from a plurimetabolic syndrome; we've already talked about it. You also told me you smoked. Are you still smoking? I feel I must insist—it's ever so important that you stop. What worries you most about giving up smoking? I see, your life hasn't been easy and a cigarette

makes you feel better. Have you ever been treated for depression? Years ago, you took antidepressants for a certain period, but you are feeling quite well at the moment. I suggest we start a treatment, the same you tried ten years ago, when you stopped smoking for about three weeks. Yes, nicotine patches. Last time you stopped them too quickly. I know, they are quite expensive, but cigarettes are not free. Let's fix an appointment for next week. How about that? Good—I am pleased you trust me."

First visit for cessation

"Right, here we are. Could you please fill in these two tests? One is to assess your degree of dependence, the other concerns your mood, since you are a bit sensitive from this point of view. Right. We have a score of seven from the Fagerström test, and the other shows a very slight form of depression, but don't worry about it. I suggest you follow a treatment course based on nicotine substitution. You are worried about having to stop smoking as soon as we apply the patch, as the leaflet says? Well, in that case we can really say that the leaflet contains a half-lie: you can continue smoking even when the patch is on. Obviously it is better to stop immediately, but if you don't feel you can, you may give up gradually. Do you feel more happy about it now? Agreed. You will put a patch on, the one with the highest nicotine content and continue smoking freely. But use this little trick: before lighting a cigarette ask yourself if you really cannot go without. If the answer is yes, postpone lighting that cigarette; if not, just light it. Do this with every cigarette, without forcing it. You will feel the effect of the patch in making the wish for a cigarette progressively weaker. See you in 7 days' time and you can tell me. Feel free to phone me if you feel things are difficult, but I am sure you will not have any problems whatsoever."

A common practical problem: stop immediately or gradually?

There are different answers to this question. We believe the approach with the patient improves, and consequently the probabilities of success also improve, if the treatment suggested manages to make him feel a decrease in the need to smoke. In order to achieve this, the patient must be initially left free to smoke, planning the quitting day at the second or third visit. A reasonable lapse of time from the start to the quitting day is usually 7-10 days; longer is not advantageous, since this would negatively influence the patient's motivation. This approach makes it possible to overcome, especially in heavy smokers, the terror caused by the idea of giving up smoking there and then. Obviously if you have a patient who has decided himself that he will stop that day or who has already stopped the day before, it becomes crucial not to miss the opportunity giving as much support as possible with treatment, and treatment will be better if based on nicotine.

You might wonder whether an increase in the level of nicotine in the blood may be harmful for the lady in this case. Well, it is by far the lesser of two evils. All specialists in tobacco addiction agree that a form of "accompaniment" toward cessation with nicotine patches should be seriously considered in patients who are very much afraid of failing. Remember that self-efficacy ("I think I shall make it") is our guiding light. In this case, I thought about nicotine patches because they had worked in the past, even if only partially, and because the patient had a history of significant clinical depression. We could have opted for bupropion, but I preferred to use patches. Let's now see how it worked.

Second visit for cessation

"Good morning, Mrs. Smith. How did things go? You are smoking only six cigarettes a day? What? You aren't satisfied? You've been very good indeed—I hadn't asked you to stop smoking completely. You noticed a marked decrease in the urge to smoke in the morning. Good! Excellent observation! The urge to smoke as soon as you wake up is the classical picture of nicotine dependence. This means that the patch is doing its job. So, can we think about taking this big step forward now? Well, you choose the day. Tomorrow is perfect. Ah, yes, the gesture ... I suggest you use nicotine inhalers. No, not instead of the patch, but in addition to it. You will keep the inhaler in your mouth, starting from tomorrow, recharging it when you get the impression you can no longer taste anything. Do not inhale as if it were a cigarette. It is not dangerous, but it tends to irritate your throat. You should suck the inhaler as if it were a pipe, and it will help you get over the more difficult moments, even if it will be the patch that will give the most support. Is everything clear? Very well, see you in a week's time and ... good luck!"

It will be very useful for this patient too to activate a buddy or support by phone, extremely important during the first week of cessation. Combined nicotine substitution treatment increases support to the patient a great deal.

Third visit

"So here we are; I see you are smiling, Mrs. Smith. It was better than you expected. It was difficult at times ... but only for brief moments. Very, very good! Things couldn't have gone better. Now, all we have to do is continue like this, without changing anything. You don't change a winning team.

You are worried because your appetite has increased. Yes, this is an effect of giving up smoking, but let's remain concentrated on the smoking, just try to eat more fruit and vegetables and exercise a little more. No, Mrs. Smith, I won't put you on a diet, not now. We'll discuss it in 2 weeks' time at the next visit. Phone me if you need to, and ... congratulations!"

I purposely did not put Mrs. Smith on a diet because it would have been pointless. It would have just added more responsibility and would have discouraged her, since it is often useless at this stage; briefly it would have undermined her confidence. "Face one thing at a time!" English authors say. The increase in weight during cessation must be dealt with, when it occurs, as a controlled fall.

Fourth visit

"Right, so here we are again. You haven't smoked for three weeks. Other people smoking start to annoy you, but at times your own desire to smoke is still quite strong. Yes, that's normal, we are still only half way; we've finished the most difficult part. Surprised? Your appetite is still bigger than it used to be, but you've stopped putting on weight ... only three kilos. Good—this is a good sign. You'll lose these three kilos in the course of the next few months. A diet at this stage would be pointless. Try to exercise more, it will also help reduce the tension. You feel very proud—good! Don't worry about when the time to get rid of the patch or the inhalers comes: we'll do it gradually and not before a month's time. Everything is going very well, we are exactly where we should be. See you in three weeks' time. No changes in the treatment."

It is important to reassure the patient about the transitory effect of nicotine-based treatment but, at the same time, to urge him not to be in a hurry to reduce the dosages. In the combined treatment, the patches follow the classical pattern; whereas the additional treatment is decided on by the patient in a personalized manner: sometimes it is almost ignored, whereas other times it is used extensively. It is worth backing the patient's decisions at this stage, trying to correct him gradually in the following visits.

Fifth visit

"You haven't smoked since 26th September? Good heavens, that's six weeks—the number of cigarettes you haven't smoked is more than

1000! Surprised? Well, you used to smoke 25 cigarettes a day, and you stopped smoking 42 days ago ... I know it seems impossible! A thousand really is a lot, a 100 metre rope! You've been very good. A lot of people tell you so? It's a great satisfaction, isn't it? Now we can start reducing the patches. You'll move on to the intermediate dosage for two weeks, then on to the lower one for another two weeks. Then—stop. You can continue using the inhalers as you wish. I'll see you in five weeks' time, when you have finished treatment. I don't think you will notice the reduction, but phone me if you feel you are in difficulty."

The reduction of substitution treatment is not usually noticed. Sometimes patients tend to overdo it: they forget to apply the patches and, since they do not feel any immediate negative effects, they tend to test themselves by suspending treatment. The worsening of their condition tends to be, in these cases, devious and mostly involves the patient's mood (short temper, depressed mood, etc.) with a consequent increase in the desire to smoke.

Sixth visit

"Right. So this is our last appointment, as far as smoking is concerned, I mean. Don't worry about those who have started smoking again after years of not smoking. You certainly must know a lot of people who have never lit a cigarette again after quitting and who have no intention of doing so, even if they still feel like a cigarette sometimes. The gradual cessation of the patches went according to the normal plan, but you still keep an inhaler in your mouth even if you recharge it every 2-3 days. Um, you still have 6-7 refills. No, that's not a problem, it's just that from now on it could become a habit. I suggest you finish the remaining refills, keeping the inhaler in your mouth until you get tired of it. Ring me when you throw it away. You will stop missing it after no more than 2-3 days of nonuse, but I'd rather hear about it from you personally. Good, you have done something very important for your health—don't waste the effort you made! No, Mrs. Smith, I don't deserve any credit for it. The exact opposite is true: you deserve all the credit! I just made it easier for you. All right, let's say we have both done a good job."

Well, of course, not all cases go so well. Let's examine one where things didn't work out and some possible solutions.

7.3 Case C

First visit

"Good morning, Mr. White. The results of your blood tests are all right. I see you are quite fit even from the point of view of your weight. Do you smoke? Well, five cigarettes a day means that you smoke. You are right, you do not have any other risk factors, you practice sports regularly, that's true, but I have to point out that with smoking there is no level of safety. No, I don't want to join your family in reproaching you, I would only like you to give me the opportunity to help you give up. Even five cigarettes a day (and sometimes it's ten) can make you addicted. You don't really believe so ... Well, let's put it to the test with this specific assessment. Right, done—now let's see ... Yes, in actual fact your Fagerström test score is zero, but this doesn't rule out that you may have a psychological dependence, which is sometimes more devious than the physical dependence of heavy smokers. I know you have stopped smoking more than once, but have always started again and that the last time you gave up was five years ago. All right, I'll accept your promise to stop smoking tomorrow, even if I don't agree with the fact that you will be doing it to stop me worrying: you should be doing it for yourself and for those who love you. Shall we meet in seven days' time to see how things are going? No, it's not too early—a simple 10-minute visit. Yes, I'd rather do it this way. See you soon."

Even if, in theory, these cases characterized by a limited number of cigarettes and by a negative FTND test appear to be less complex than the previous ones, this is not always true. The strong ambivalence is characterised by a low priority of cessation, by the false idea that "I can stop when I decide to." Treatment is not very useful. The guidelines do not recommend treatment in light smokers, although in our surgery we tend to prescribe it even in these cases. It certainly does not have such an important role as it had in the cases we described above.

Second visit

"So, how did this week without smoking go? You didn't smoke at all. Ah, you smoked two cigarettes on Sunday and one yesterday. You say you smoked in very particular situations. Bear in mind that in order not to want to smoke, you mustn't smoke; otherwise you keep the desire alive and sooner or later you will go back to your daily cigarettes. You are not convinced. All right, let's consider yesterday's cigarette and the two on Sunday a mistake. I'll

see you again in two weeks' time and we will evaluate this attempt in a better way."

As you can see there is no point in insisting or in suggesting treatment: if you confront resistances firmly, you end up by making them even stronger.

Third visit

"How are you getting on with your smoking? You are pleased because you are only smoking one cigarette a day, always at the same time, and your family hasn't discovered it. It is certainly a step in the right direction, but you still haven't stopped. No, I am not saying that one cigarette a day is terribly bad for you, though it certainly doesn't do you any good; I am just saying that you haven't stopped. Let's meet in two weeks' time—all right, three, but let's meet to see how things are going."

In these cases the smoker's attitude is to minimize the problem, which is a psychological reaction to the realization that he has failed. The patient realizes he is incapable of total control, but he does not want to admit it, and pointing it out does not shift the balance in the right direction. The therapist's attitude should be understanding; he should not judge, but be persuasive, trying to avoid any possible dispute with the patient. A useful point in these cases is to recommend that the patient avoid alcohol completely; alcohol, even at low doses, plays a strategic role in light smokers, both by enhancing craving, otherwise very slight or absent in these patients, and by weakening the feeling of behavior control. It is important for the therapist to remember the patient's initial motivations, even if weak, and to play on them.

Fourth visit

"What's wrong, Mr. White? I see you are irritated. I understand, you are in a hurry because you have a lot of business engagements. On the other hand, as your doctor, I believe giving up smoking is extremely important for you. So, you are smoking three, sometimes five, cigarettes a day and you are no longer prepared to listen to your family's complaints ... or to mine. I see. You say we have chosen a bad time. That might be. Let's see how you get on in the next few months. We are at the end of October. Try to plan giving up smoking as a New Year's resolution. You think it is an excellent idea? Good: new year, new life, is what they say. Mark it on your calendar today. I am quite prepared to give you a hand when you decide to take this important step. Let me know. No problem, goodbye."

Why this suggestion to give up as of the first of January? Because that has been considered to be the decisive option in giving up smoking for 16,000 English people who stopped smoking, in a study carried out by Robert West (one of the world's greatest experts on smoking addiction) a few years ago. We do not know if they were heavy smokers, if they had anxiety problems, or if they drank alcohol; all we know is that to quit on New Year's day was a plus for them. It should therefore be borne in mind, especially when no other options or resources are available.

I would like at this stage to briefly discuss unconventional anti-smoking treatment.

Many different forms of unconventional treatment have been suggested. Some have also been validated, such as hypnosis, even if they have limited availability and effect; others carry a more controversial validation or have not been validated at all, such as acupuncture. Still others, even if used a lot, have no specific scientific basis, such as homeopathy, or, even worse, spirit healing. Personally I have used, and still do sometimes, auriculotherapy (a sort of acupuncture) for the cessation of smoking and have often had positive experiences with it. This evaluation has not, however, been confirmed by scientific research, and therefore I do not feel I can recommend it. We have all met smokers, even heavy smokers, who have stopped smoking with electrical shocks, herb teas, or other atypical solutions. This does not mean that we should suggest approaches that do not have any scientific validation. Tobacco addiction is a normal mental disorder which in addition carries a high morbidity and mortality rate, and as such should be treated no differently from other disorders. On the other hand, I do not suggest you interfere with a patient who is successfully giving up smoking with acupuncture; he must be encouraged to continue with his attempt, but you should make yourself available to reassess the situation if the cessation process does not have a positive outcome.

7.4 Searching for a Guiding Idea

We are still missing something—something that can be remembered, a direction to be followed. We are missing the "guiding idea." But we already have it, you might say. We have hypertension, dyslipidemia, gastritis, recurrent pneumonia, asthma attacks, etc. Who would want more reference points than these? You are right; from a rational point of view your observation is faultless. Pity, though, that it often does not work, does not produce the desired results. No, I am not saying that patients are not interested in their health, absolutely not. I am pointing out that in addictions rationality loses when faced with emotions. Smokers are more receptive to emotional communication than to professional communication.

And emotional communication is made up of verbal and body language, of facial expressions and allegories, of facts mixed with images. It is a kind of language that directly addresses the amygdala of our brain, our "emotional microprocessor," the part of our brain that quickly mediates our learning of what we like and fixes it in our memory, often in an indelible manner and usually by associating this memory with images, sounds, sensations, "flashes"—in other words, Proust's madeleine cake which evokes in him the desire to search for lost time. Psychological dependence on smoking follows the same paths, when certain situations, apparently insignificant or routine, set off in the ex-smoker a strong craving for a cigarette.

And so we need a guiding idea, an indelible image that will last for months, sometimes for years.

I know, it sounds peculiar, but I can assure you it isn't. If you allow yourself to be involved a bit at a time in an understanding style of dialogue with the patients who are giving up smoking, the similes, the images will start to flow freely in the exchange and to your surprise your patient will start saying things like,

> *"Doctor, do you know what struck me most when you asked me to stop smoking a month ago? The description you gave of my life wasting away like a cigarette, leaving only ashes. It was like an electric shock!"*

The objection could be: but surgeries around the whole world are full of similar images; prevention campaigns have been set up, but not with any great result, apparently.

True, you find the same images on posters and leaflets, but the guiding idea is born between you and your patient, it is your, his image. It is born out of understanding dialogue, out of the identification with the patient's conflicts. It is inside him and you make it surface. How? By giving free play to the images, the examples:

> *"How can I explain this? It's as if they freed you from a collar and chain,"*

for example, when you are talking about addiction.

Many images are yours and remain simple examples, useful but not particularly significant. Other images go down deeper, almost as if they were passwords, and open up pathways. And they are remembered:

> *"Do you remember, Doctor, when you told me that with my asthma, lighting a cigarette is like a killer putting a pillow over the victim's face to suffocate him? Well, when I feel having like a cigarette I always think about that picture ... and I no longer feel like having one."*

There are thousands of examples, and they come to mind as small flash-images during conversation. Sometimes they come to mind while you are explaining a concept to the patient, sometimes while the patient is speaking and you throw them back at him like arrows:

- "*Sometimes my wife complains about the smell of cigarettes, she sends me away ...*"
- "*She says she doesn't want to lick an ashtray.*"
- "*Oh, yes, how disgusting!*"

I don't want to make a list, it's pointless. What I want to make you understand is that you must rely upon these images, use them constantly; and when you see from your patient's expression that they have made an impact on him, he has probably found his guiding idea. All this might sound a bit like nursery school, but on the other hand, addiction is a memory disorder.

Group Therapy

Fabio Lugoboni [1]

[1] Department of Internal Medicine, Medical Unit for Addictive Disorders, University of Verona, Policlinico GB Rossi, Verona, Italy

In order to give a complete picture, we cannot forget that in developed countries one of the forms of treatment most frequently offered to smokers who intend to give up smoking is group therapy. Group therapy is of many different kinds, from support groups (smokers who have given up smoking who find renewed energy helping other smokers not to relapse, or who feel it is their duty to make what they have learnt and the intuitions they have had available to others) that follow the model of Alcoholics Anonymous, to therapy groups run by volunteers who are themselves ex-smokers or by professionals. In these latter cases, the groups may be closed, when a group starts off with a certain number of smokers and ends at a pre-established date; semi-open, when a closed group may be joined by a limited and controlled number of smokers during its course of action; or open, as in the case of support groups where attendance is free and the duration may be indefinite. The complexity, for those who are running the groups, increases the more open the group is; and the therapist's ability consists in giving importance to the ex-smokers' experiences in favor of the new entries, knowing, however, how to intervene in a decisive manner in the case of a senior member of the group relapsing.

The strong point of the various types of groups lies in the fact that they are based on cooperation, which tends to produce enthusiasm in those who have given up smoking in this way and in those who run the groups. They are also cheap, and reach a considerable number of smokers. The weak point, often not realized or not admitted, is selection: complex smokers tend to refuse the offer of group therapy. Another negative point, particularly concerning closed groups run by therapists, is having to wait for admission; sometimes you are kept on stand-by for months because, for example, a group has just started and will last for three months, thus postponing the setting up of a new group until four months later. It is a bit like guided museum tours, but obviously with much longer time intervals. All this waiting, as we have seen and will examine more deeply in the second part, is very bad for the motivation process. It is, however, important that the experience of group therapy should be assessed by the general practitioners among the associated doctors working together and sharing the premises. The possibility of reinforcing or combining the forms of treatment described above with group therapy, run by a doctor of the associated group who is either more sensitive to the problem or more prepared to be involved, or the possibility of delegating a nurse to do it, since nurses are traditionally more inclined and trained for interaction with the patient, opens up interesting innovative scenarios and is potentially able to attract attention and financial incentives.

How to Avoid Relapses

Fabio Lugoboni [1]

[1] Department of Internal Medicine, Medical Unit for Addictive Disorders, University of Verona, Policlinico GB Rossi, Verona, Italy

Even though you will find a more in-depth analysis on preventing relapses in Part II, it is important to discuss some basic concepts here; they are an integral part of our basic training. Since smoking is a form of addiction, it is by definition a chronic relapsing disease; relapses are therefore frequent events after cessation of smoking and produce, in almost all cases, a return to the previous smoking habits. The speed of this return is generally faster, the higher the Fagerström test score at the moment when the decision to give up smoking was made. Thus it can be expected that subjects with low scores will still be smoking, though in an inconstant manner, 4-6 weeks after the relapse; whereas those with high FTND scores will tend, after only a few days, to resume smoking the same number of cigarettes they used to smoke. All this can be easily explained by the phenomenon of pharmacological tolerance to nicotine, as happens with all addiction-inducing drugs. If a heavy smoker, after having stopped smoking for a month, lights a cigarette, he will probably feel just as dizzy as the youngster who smokes his first cigarette; the difference is in the speed at which he will get used to the following drags. In order to avoid this risk, it is important to help the patient recognize that it is not so much the outside situation that leads to the relapse, as what happens inside himself ("I risk starting to smoke again not so much because I am at a dinner where a lot of people are smoking, but because deep down I am willing to be offered a cigarette or to ask for one!"). He also needs to know that oaths or binding commitments with oneself or with one's family are of no use; the more the quitting is emphasized, the more difficult the recovery becomes in the case of a relapse. This paradoxical phenomenon is called the abstinence violation effect (AVE), and occurs when giving up smoking has involved personal prestige, a solemn commitment, a vow, an oath, etc. The relapse, which might be represented by a single cigarette smoked when not totally sober, produces such a strong emotional backlash that self-esteem goes to pieces and devaluing thoughts about oneself are triggered—for example, "I am a weakling, I am worthless." "There is no hope for me, I am condemned to smoke all my life."—leading the smoker to find comfort in smoking and in the fact that smoking can modulate one's mood. Such a subject will tend to start smoking again quickly and will be more difficult to reclaim.

This is why it is important to recommend to our patient on finishing treatment that he contact us immediately if he should light a cigarette. If you are a general practitioner, frequent contacts with the patient or his family will allow you to send quick, but extremely useful, motivational "flashes," aimed at giving high consideration to the abstinence he has achieved, and at weighing the stimuli to smoking correctly. Time, as you know, tends to work in the opposite direction.

10 The Problem of Weight Increase

Fabio Lugoboni [1]

[1] Department of Internal Medicine, Medical Unit for Addictive Disorders, University of Verona, Policlinico GB Rossi, Verona, Italy

A varying increase in body weight occurs in 85% of the patients who give up smoking. This occurs mainly for four reasons: loss of the anorectic action of nicotine, lowering of basal metabolism, slow but definite improvement in the perception of the taste of food no longer reduced by smoking, and marked compensatory orality: the patient constantly feels the need to put something into his mouth, preferably sweets, for self-gratification.

Since the fear of putting on weight is present in practically all younger smokers and in female smokers, it is important to remind the patient that a weight gain is quite likely, but is limited and temporary. The increase in weight can be effectively limited by drinking a lot of water and eating more fruit and vegetables, avoiding alcohol for some time, thus also achieving an important effect on the desire to smoke. One should in fact remember that alcohol is a powerful stimulant to craving, and we ask all our patients to avoid drinking. It is not a good idea for overweight patients to start a diet at the same time that they give up smoking. Patients suffering from heart conditions or diabetes who put on weight need particularly careful reassuring and explaining that the risk connected to this increase is widely counterbalanced by the reduction of the risks induced by smoking. Female smokers need to be told that the esthetic problem of putting on weight is easily counterbalanced by several positive effects immediately visible (skin color, the fact they no longer smell of cigarette smoke, progressive reduction of wrinkles), and that mostly it is temporary.

11 The Patient Who Does not Want to Try to Give up Smoking

Fabio Lugoboni [1]

[1] Department of Internal Medicine, Medical Unit for Addictive Disorders, University of Verona, Policlinico GB Rossi, Verona, Italy

The patients who do not even want to try to give up smoking might not be sufficiently informed about the damages caused by smoking, not be motivated to quit, be demoralized by previous attempts, or suffer from basal depression. The doctor's role should be governed by an approach built on the "5Rs" (Figure 10). They are:

- **Relevance**: Very detailed information should be presented on the importance of giving up smoking, specific to the patient's health conditions or to his family's (for example, children).
- **Risks**: The doctor should help the patient identify the negative consequences smoking has for him personally, such as breathing problems, frequent bronchitis, teeth disorders, etc.; and longer-term damages which are bound to be relevant to the patient, such as cancer, heart attacks, and strokes in the family or in acquaintances.
- **Rewards**: The doctor should lead the patient to recognize the undoubted advantages obtained by giving up smoking, e.g., health, environmental hygiene, self-esteem, cost savings, etc.
- **Roadblocks**: Being very understanding, one should invite the patient to identify the main obstacles to an anti-smoking treatment, e.g., abstinence symptoms, problems connected to his environment, fear of putting on weight, depression, fear of failing, etc.
- **Repetition**: All the stages of treatment should be repeated every time you see the patient again.

Before you start, if you decide to, on the more technical part (which can be read even if you do not have specific pharmacological knowledge), I would like to end with a recommendation:

> **Resistances (recognize them in order not to reinforce them)**
>
> - Challenge (attack on the doctor's statements)
> - Disconfirmation (questioning the competence of the doctor)
> - Attack on the doctor's honesty
> - Inattention
> - Inappropriate answers
> - Talk over the doctor
> - Interrupting abruptly
> - Silence

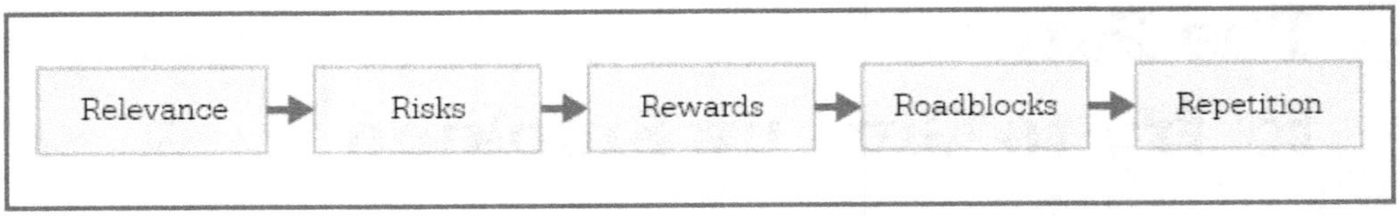

Figure 10. "5Rs" scheme for smoking patient [Fiore, 2008]

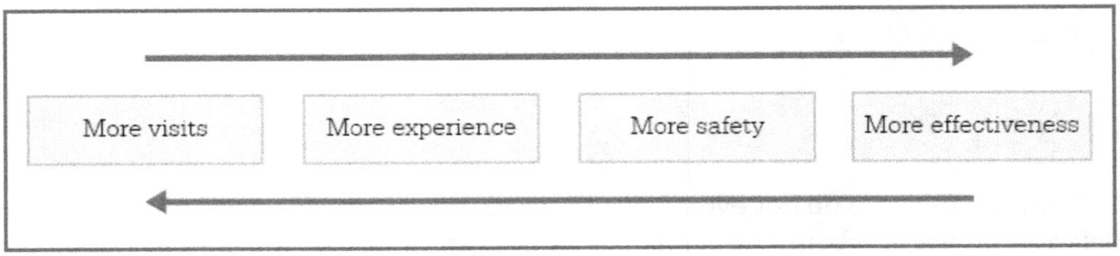

Figure 11. Virtuous circle

once again, try to treat and follow your smoker patients. If you have got this far, it means that the subject holds some interest for you. So what is stopping you from starting to treat them? If you don't try, you will never know. There is, however, no half way of doing it: "I'll give you the medication and then phone me," or "Try your best and if you have difficulties phone me." If you behave like this you will not achieve appreciable and long-lasting results and therefore you will not get any satisfaction and "reinforcement" out of it (Figure 11). Clever you, you have understood what I mean: just like a cigarette.

References

- Fiore MC, Jaén CR, Baker TB, et al. Treating tobacco use and dependence: 2008 update. U.S. Department of Health and Human Services. Public Health Service, 2008

Part II

THE THEORY

12 Smoking and Health

Fabio Lugoboni [1]

[1] Department of Internal Medicine, Medical Unit for Addictive Disorders, University of Verona, Policlinico GB Rossi, Verona, Italy

Almost all the books that address the issue of smoking begin by describing the damage from smoke. As mentioned at the beginning of this book, we have chosen not to do that. This does not mean that the argument goes away, somehow, neglected or snubbed. We will do it here, in depth medically, and we will do it in a concise, streamlined manner (Table XII). Data on the harmful effects of smoking will be briefly reported, with related references.

- Smoking is the leading cause of avoidable death in developed countries [World Health Organization, 2003].
- Tobacco will kill more than 175 million people worldwide between 2005 and 2030 [Shafey, 2009].
- Tobacco use costs the world hundreds of billions of dollars each year [World Health Organization, 2008].
- Half of all tobacco-related deaths occur during the active years of life. Exposure to secondhand smoke costs the U.S. $10 billion annually in medical costs and lost productivity. There is no safe level of smoke [World Health Organization, 2006].
- The inability to curb the use of cigarettes is the worst failure in the history of preventive medicine [Blum, 2004].
- Cigarette smoking increases by 50% the rate of absenteeism among workers [Jackson, 2007].

In Italy [data from DOXA, 2012]	In the world [data from WHO, 2000]
• 20.8% of adults • 24.6% of males and 17.2% of females • 70,000 deaths/year (one out of six deaths is related to smoking, or one death every 6.5 minutes)	• 1,260,000,000 smokers (1/3 of world population aged > 15) • 47% of males and 12% of females • 3,500,000 deaths/year (10,000 every day) • 10,000,000 estimated victims in 2030

Table XII. Smoking: the dimensions of the problem

- Employer-based cost/benefit of quitting smoking for 12 months, related to the likelihood of therapeutic success and weighted to the initial treatment costs (in U.S. $): varenicline: $541; bupropion: $270; placebo: $82 [Jackson, 2007].
- Programs for smoking cessation and relapse prevention for pregnant women: for every dollar invested $3 is saved in health care costs [Ruger, 2008].
- Quitting smoking has led to a decline in deaths three times higher than that obtained from blood pressure reduction and seven times higher than that obtained by reducing cholesterol levels of blood (England and Galles 1981-2000) [Unal, 2005].
- Smoking increases the risk of sudden cardiac death up to five times [Willett, 1987].
- Those who smoke 20 or more cigarettes per day increase their risk of stroke 2-4 times [Goldstein, 2011].
- Smokers have a worse functional prognosis after stroke than nonsmokers [Ovbiagele, 2006].
- The risk of death from coronary disease is greater in smokers by 70%, and 200% higher in heavy smokers. The risk of fatal myocardial infarction is four times higher in smokers than nonsmokers. Quitting smoking is associated with a drastic reduction of rehospitalization and admission into intensive care for patients post-myocardial infarction [Shopland, 1983].
- The risk of MI or stroke decreases by approximately 50% within the first two years after cessation [Ockene, 1997].
- Smoking cessation after a MI or after bypass surgery reduces the risk of death by 36% [Critchley, 2003].
- By 24 hours after cessation of smoking, a complete recovery from agonist-induced endothelial vasodilation is observed [Moreno, 1998].
- Platelet aggregation is significantly improved by 4.2 weeks following cessation of smoking [Morita, 2005].
- Coronary endothelial dysfunction is significantly improved by six months following the cessation of smoking [Hosokawa, 2008].
- HDL/LDL ratio is improved significantly by 4 weeks following cessation. [Erguder, 2006].
- Smoking increases in a linear manner the risk of abdominal aortic aneurysm [Lederle, 2003].
- Smoking doubles the risk of intermittent claudication [Willigendael, 2005].
- Smoking greatly reduces the benefit of good blood pressure control [Journath, 2005].
- Smoking reduces the benefit of statins [Milionis, 2001].
- Smoking is associated with a significantly increased risk of diabetes mellitus, which is 79% higher even in light smokers [Wannamethee, 2001].
- Smoking is associated with an increased risk of chronic renal failure [Shankar, 2006].

- There is a documented direct relationship between the number of cigarettes smoked and the risk of developing periodontitis: under 10 cigarettes a day, three times the risk; over 30 a day, six times the risk [Tomar, 2000].
- Smoking is associated with a 70% increased risk of fetal death [Yuan, 2005].
- Smoking less than ten cigarettes per day is associated with a 60% increase of premature births; smoking more than ten a day increases the risk by 90% [Burguet, 2004].
- Smoking is associated with a 60% increase in female infertility [Augood, 1998].
- Smoking is associated with a 3-year premature menopause [Kinney, 2006].
- The risk of ischemic stroke for users of oral contraceptives is four times greater in smokers [Kemmeren, 2002].
- Smoking increases the risk of COPD (chronic obstructive pulmonary disease), acute bronchitis, pneumonia, and influenza [American Thoracic Society, 1996].
- Smoking is by far the leading cause of lung cancer, with an RR of 20 [Wald, 1996].
- Smoking is the major cause of cancers of the larynx, esophagus, stomach, liver, pancreas, bladder, kidney, uterus, and blood [U.S. Department of Health and Human Services, 2004].
- Smoking is associated with loss of bone mineral density and subsequent osteoporosis, and is a cofactor of spontaneous fractures [Rapuri, 2000].
- Smoking causes a 40% increase in the risk of cataracts and three times increased risk of macular degeneration [Fagerström, 2002].
- Although the greatest benefits are obtained in young smokers, it is greatly worth stopping at any age and any comorbidity [Brunnhuber, 2007].
- Smokers in poor countries get sick more and die earlier than the smokers in rich countries [World Health Organization, 2004].
- In Bangladesh, among the poorest households, ten times more is spent on tobacco than on schools. In Egypt, in families with low incomes, spending on tobacco is more than 10% of the household budget [Efroymson, 2001].
- Tobacco harms the environment: pesticides and fertilizers damage the soil; firewood for drying tobacco is a cause of deforestation; cigarettes cause thousands of fires and great loss of life every year [World Bank, 2005].
- 200,000 hectares of forest are destroyed every year to make way for tobacco plantations, mainly in the Third World [Geist, 1999].

References

- American Thoracic Society. Cigarette smoking and health. *Am J Respir Crit Care Med* 1996; 153: 861-5

- Augood C, Duckitt K, Templeton AA. Smoking and female infertility: a systematic review and meta-analysis. *Hum Reprod* 1998; 13: 1532-9
- Blum A, Solberg E, Wolinsky H. The Surgeon General's report on smoking and health 40 years later: still wandering in the desert. *Lancet* 2004; 363: 97-8
- Brunnhuber C, Cummings KM, Feit S, et al. Putting evidence into practice: Smoking Cessation, BMJ Report 2007
- Burguet A, Kaminski M, Abraham-Lerat L, et al; EPIPAGE Study Group. The complex relationship between smoking in pregnancy and very preterm delivery. Results of the Epipage Study. *Br J Obstet Gynaecol* 2004; 111: 258-65
- Critchley J, Capewell S. Smoking cessation for the secondary prevention of coronary heart disease. *Cochrane Database Syst Rev* 2003; (4): CD003041
- Efroymson D, Ahmed S, Townsend J, et al. Hungry for tobacco: an analysis of the economic impact of tobacco consumption on the poor in Bangladesh. *Tobacco Control* 2001; 10: 212-7
- Ergüder IB, Ergüder T, Ozkan C, et al. Short-term effects of smoking cessation on blood antioxidant parameters and paraoxonase activity in healthy asymptomatic long-term cigarette smokers. *Inhal Toxicol* 2006; 18: 575-9
- Fagerström K. The epidemiology of smoking: health consequences and benefits of cessation. *Drugs* 2002; 62 (Suppl 2): 1-9
- Geist HJ. Global assessment of deforestation related to tobacco farming. *Tob Control* 1999; 8: 18-28
- Goldstein LB, Bushnell CD, Adams RJ, et al; American Heart Association Stroke Council; Council on Cardiovascular Nursing; Council on Epidemiology and Prevention; Council for High Blood Pressure Research; Council on Peripheral Vascular Disease, and Interdisciplinary Council on Quality of Care and Outcomes Research. Guidelines for the primary prevention of stroke: a guideline for healthcare professionals from the American Heart Association/American Stroke Association. *Stroke* 2011; 42: 517-54
- Hosokawa S, Hiasa Y, Miyazaki S, et al. Effects of smoking cessation on coronary endothelial function in patients with recent myocardial infarction. *Int J Cardiol* 2008; 128: 48-52
- Jackson KC 2nd, Nahoopii R, Said Q, et al. An employer-based cost-benefit analysis of a novel pharmacotherapy agent for smoking cessation. *J Occup Environ Med* 2007; 49: 453-60
- Journath G, Nilsson PM, Petersson U, et al. Hypertensive smokers have a worse cardiovascular risk profile than non-smokers in spite of treatment--a national study in Sweden. *Blood Press* 2005; 14: 144-50
- Kemmeren JM, Tanis BC, van den Bosch MA, et al. Risk of Arterial Thrombosis in Relation to Oral Contraceptives (RATIO) study: oral contraceptives and the risk of ischemic stroke. *Stroke* 2002; 33: 1202-8
- Kinney A, Kline J, Levin B. Alcohol, caffeine and smoking in relation to age at menopause. *Maturitas* 2006; 54: 27-38
- Lederle FA, Nelson DB, Joseph AM. Smokers' relative risk for aortic aneurysm compared with other smoking-related diseases: a systematic review. *J Vasc Surg* 2003; 38: 329-34

- Milionis HJ, Rizos E, Mikhailidis DP. Smoking diminishes the beneficial effect of statins: observations from the landmark trials. *Angiology* 2001; 52: 575-87
- Moreno H Jr, Chalon S, Urae A, et al. Endothelial dysfunction in human hand veins is rapidly reversible after smoking cessation. *Am J Physiol* 1998; 275: H1040-5
- Morita H, Ikeda H, Haramaki N, et al. Only two-week smoking cessation improves platelet aggregability and intraplatelet redox imbalance of long-term smokers. *J Am Coll Cardiol* 2005; 45: 589-94
- Ockene IS, Miller NH. Cigarette smoking, cardiovascular disease, and stroke: a statement for healthcare professionals from the American Heart Association. American Heart Association Task Force on Risk Reduction. *Circulation* 1997; 96: 3243-7
- Ovbiagele B, Weir CJ, Saver JL, et al; IMAGES Investigators. Effect of smoking status on outcome after acute ischemic stroke. *Cerebrovasc Dis* 2006; 21: 260-5
- Rapuri PB, Gallagher JC, Balhorn KE, et al. Smoking and bone metabolism in elderly women. *Bone* 2000; 27: 429-36
- Ruger JP, Emmons KM. Economic evaluations of smoking cessation and relapse prevention programs for pregnant women: a systematic review. *Value Health* 2008; 11: 180-90
- Shafey O, Eriksen M, Ross H, et al. The Tobacco Atlas, Third Edition. The American Cancer Society, 2009
- Shankar A, Klein R, Klein BE. The association among smoking, heavy drinking, and chronic kidney disease. *Am J Epidemiol* 2006; 164: 263-71
- Shopland DR. The health consequences of smoking: cardiovascular disease. A report of the Surgeon General. United States: Public Health Service. Office of the Surgeon General, 1983
- Tomar SL, Asma S. Smoking-attributable periodontitis in the United States: findings from NHANES III. National Health and Nutrition Examination Survey. *J Periodontal* 2000; 71: 743-51
- Unal B, Critchley JA, Capewell S. Modelling the decline in coronary heart disease deaths in England and Wales, 1981-2000: comparing contributions from primary prevention and secondary prevention. *BMJ* 2005; 331: 614
- U.S. Department of Health and Human Services. The health consequences of smoking: what it means to you. U.S. Department of Health and Human Services, Centers for Disease Control and Prevention, National Center for Chronic Disease Prevention and Health Promotion, Office on Smoking and Health, 2004
- Wald NJ, Hackshaw AK. Cigarette smoking: an epidemiological overview. *Br Med Bull* 1996; 52: 3-11
- Wannamethee SG, Shaper AG, Perry IJ; British Regional Heart Study. Smoking as a modifiable risk factor for type 2 diabetes in middle-aged men. *Diabetes Care* 2001; 24: 1590-5
- Willett WC, Green A, Stampfer MJ, et al. Relative and absolute excess risks of coronary heart disease among women who smoke cigarettes. *N Engl J Med* 1987; 317: 1303-9
- Willigendael EM, Teijink JA, Bartelink ML, et al. Smoking and the patency of lower extremity bypass grafts: a meta-analysis. *J Vasc Surg* 2005; 42: 67-74
- World Bank. *Promot Educ* 2005; (Suppl 4): 12-55

- World Health Organization. Report on the Global Tobacco Epidemic. Geneva: WHO, 2008
- World Health Organization. The cost attributable to tobacco use. Geneva: WHO, 2006
- World Health Organization. The World Health Report. Geneva: WHO, 2003
- World Health Organization. World no tobacco day 2004 materials. Geneva: WHO, 2004
- Yuan H, Platt RW, Morin L, et al. Fetal deaths in the United States, 1997 vs 1991. *Am J Obstet Gynecol* 2005; 93: 489-95

13 Neurochemical Addiction

Cristiano Chiamulera [1]

[1] Associate Professor of Pharmacology, Department of Medicine and Public Health, Verona University, Italy

13.1 The Psychoactive Effects of Nicotine

Smoking causes a number of changes in mood, attention, and emotion. These pleasant psychological effects determine the onset and maintenance of compulsive behavior persisting over time [Heishman, 1994]. Similarly, nicotine induces improvement of cognitive processes, the ability to concentrate, attention, and psychomotor performance. Smokers report anxiolytic effects and improved mood. These positive effects increase the likelihood of continuing to smoke and are related by recent MRI studies to metabolic activation by nicotine of brain areas such as the amygdala, thalamus, and nucleus accumbens (NACC), known for their involvement in affective processes. Smoking is therefore the chronic consumption of nicotine. Smoking behavior is carefully regulated—both in frequency and intensity—in order to maintain stable plasma levels of nicotine [Corrigall, 1999]. Nicotine reaches the brain within seconds after inhalation. This is possible because the manufacturing and combustion characteristics of the cigarette make nicotine available in a form that rapidly penetrates the protective membranes of the brain. The close temporal association—it is called **contingency**—between the act of sucking and the pleasurable effects is the key to the establishment of the **reinforcing behavior** of taking the drug.

13.2 Nicotinic Receptors

Nicotine enters the brain and exerts its effects by binding directly to a known type of cholinergic receptors, called **nicotinic receptors**. They respond to acetylcholine nicotinic receptors and are involved in different physiological processes, including increased energy, alertness, and attention. They have a structure consisting of five protein subunits, which form different compositions with different functions, depending on the area of the brain where they are located (Figure 12). The protein subunits are arranged around a central channel through which pass

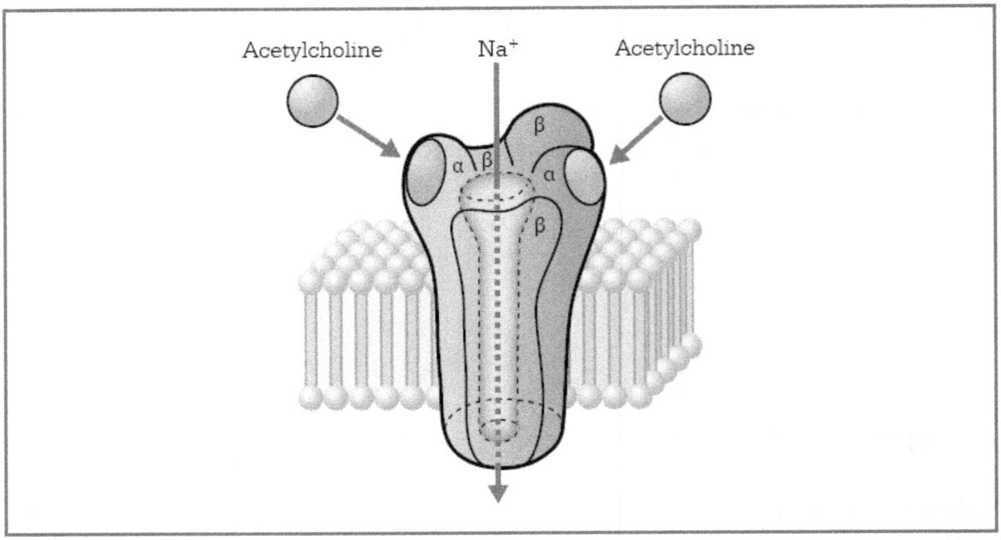

Figure 12. Schematic representation of nicotine receptor

ions Na^+ e Ca^{2+}: the binding of nicotine to the nicotinic receptor alters the flow of ions across neuronal membranes, induces a depolarization, and causes the excitation of the neuronal cell. The nine α and three β subunits known so far are able to constitute the nicotinic receptors [De Biasi, 2006]. The $\alpha_4\beta_2$ composition has been identified as the most important in mediating nicotine dependence. In fact, varenicline acts as a selective nicotinic partial agonist on these receptors, and it has been recently introduced for smoking cessation.

When the receptor binds nicotine, it changes the conformation by opening up and allowing the passage of positive ions inside the cell. After a few milliseconds it returns to its original state (closed), but it is again able to bind nicotine.

The nicotinic receptor can also become insensitive to nicotine; in this case it is called "desensitised." Nicotine reaches the synapses and it persists more than acetylcholine because it can't be hydrolyzed by the acetylcholinesterase enzyme.

Exposure to low concentrations promotes the desensitisation of the receptors, which in this state have greater affinity—but a diminished responsiveness—to nicotine [De Biasi, 2006].

13.3 Reinforcing Properties, "Pathways of Pleasure", and Dopamine

The pharmacological property that a psychoactive substance must have to induce psychological dependence is called the **reinforcing property**. Several studies have indicated that nicotine is provided with reinforcement properties, similar to those described for opiates and psychostimulants [Perkins, 1999]. Years of experimentation have shown that substances with reinforcing properties lead to repeated self-administration in laboratory animals, and that the administration is bound to drive increased levels of dopamine in the NACC. It is known that the motivation and reward processes that are activated before and during activities such as eating or mating take place under the control of **dopamine**.

These results help to confirm the hypothesis that positive reinforcement resulting from the abuse of substances is associated with increased levels of dopamine in specific brain areas, such as the NACC.

The area which has been identified as a neuroanatomical target for drugs and nicotine is the mesolimbic system, also known as the "**pathways of pleasure**."

The mesolimbic system consists of neurons in the midbrain (ventral tegmentum area) that synthesize dopamine and send their nerve projections to anterior (prefrontal cortex) and ventral (NACC) areas of the brain, generally defined as limbic for their involvement in affective processes.

The dopaminergic response to a natural reinforcement is usually of phasic type, both in activating the receptor and in the release.

Conversely, the response to drugs acts on a sensitized neural substrate, where each administration stimulates the dopamine release abnormally.

Therefore, the response in the dopaminergic substance dependence is of greater magnitude and duration than in natural reinforcers [Di Chiara, 2000].

Functional MRI studies have showed how nicotine induces in smokers metabolic activation of these brain areas [Stein, 1998]. Several studies have shown that exposure to nicotine induces, via the activation of this neuroanatomical system, increased levels of dopamine and the resulting pleasant effect and euphoria with the onset of behavioral reinforcement [Di Chiara, 2000]. The blocking of dopamine reuptake by bupropion acts in the prevention of a relapse to smoking, precisely because of its dopaminergic mechanism.

We must add that bupropion also binds to nicotinic receptors, and blocks the reuptake of norepinephrine (see Chapter 16).

13.4 The Multiple Actions of Nicotine and Neuroadaptation

Nicotine also acts on the noradrenergic system, which uses **norepinephrine** as a neurotransmitter.

Cellular bodies that synthesize norepinephrine are localized in an area of the brain base called the locus coeruleus, projecting to various other structures such as the hippocampus and amygdala. This system is involved in physiological conditions of activation and alert.

During abstinence from smoking, the cells that synthesize norepinephrine have increased and abnormal activity, causing an alteration of the alert and activation central processes to which different withdrawal symptoms are attributed.

Chronic exposure to nicotine also leads to changes in the function of serotonin. These neurochemical alterations are supposed to be the basis of symptoms such as dysphoria, anhedonia, and appetite disorders.

Self-administration studies in animal laboratories have allowed us to study the behavior of compulsive intake of nicotine with various protocols mimicking the various conditions observed in smokers.

For instance, we observed that mice trained to self-administer nicotine acquire a repetitive behavior, continued for months.

Using these models it was possible to map brain areas activated under compulsive self-administration of nicotine.

Molecules associated with gene expression were studied as markers, then molecules associated with the new synthesis process of proteins and enzymes.

Mice consuming nicotine showed a specific expression of these markers in mesolimbic system areas, showing a high probability that neuroadaptation processes may have occurred [Merlo Pich, 1997].

The neuroadaptation disease manifests itself when the conditions which induced its expression are removed.

The stop in smoking unmasks the neuroadaptation processes put in place after years of smoking.

The observable phenomena are many, **tolerance** being certainly the most studied among them. There are several mechanisms establishing tolerance to nicotine, in particular those resulting from the rapid desensitisation of nicotinic receptors after the binding of nicotine to the same receptor.

Desensitisation is a reduction in the time of activation of the receptor, a kind of "brake booster."

Thus, the activation of the receptor by means of nicotine entering rapidly into the brain is very fast.

Continuous exposure to nicotine, however, can lead to desensitisation to some subtypes of nicotinic receptors, and therefore to a state of inactivity.

The human body opposes a compensation that is an up-regulation of nicotinic receptors, with a sharp increase in the number of receptors themselves.

In smokers' brains, nicotine receptors are from 100 to 300 times more numerous than in the brains of nonsmokers [Perry, 1999]. It is possible that the **up-regulation of nicotinic receptors** is the reason for the negative actions described in smoking cessation because of the excess of activity of the endogenous neurotransmitter, acetylcholine, on these receptors.

The increased cholinergic activity would induce a state of general malaise with mood disturbance, anxiety, irritability, agitation, and sleep disorders.

The brain area which is particularly activated is the locus coeruleus, the main area of increased reactions of vigilance and alert.

The locus coeruleus cells would present an abnormally increased activity during abstinence, inducing an altered brain activation, with a series of symptoms that we found to be characteristics of the syndrome of abstinence from smoking.

Hypothetically, the research carried out suggests that the smoker takes nicotine to desensitise (functionally inactivate) his surplus nicotinic receptors and reduce the negative effects of increased cholinergic activity. It is known that the most desired cigarette of the day is the first in the morning, on waking, when the effect of the up-regulation of nicotinic receptors is more evident because of the night abstinence. It is assumed that this could also be the action mechanism of NRT characterized by long-life plasma levels, such as patches and gums, which are able to "switch off" the surplus receptors.

13.5 Molecular Genetics of Smoking

Clinical genetics is focused on the study of polymorphisms of genes that encode proteins (candidate genes) involved in nicotine addiction.

There is a significant correlation between the serotonin transporter polymorphism and the age of smoking initiation.

Similar data were obtained with polymorphisms of the dopamine-2 receptor gene.

The polymorphism for metabolic enzymes of nicotine leads to smoking: those who have a rapid metabolism are less affected by the initial unpleasant effects of smoking and tend to smoke more cigarettes. The smoker phenotype is an expression of the genetic component (genotype). Although the smoker phenotype is complex, you can find some macroareas: biological, physiological, behavioral, psychological. The overlap of these phenotypic features contributes to define the type of smoker. The complexity of smoking comes from this, but also from the variability of response to therapy and the need to individualize (tailor) the intervention.

13.6 Conclusion

A better understanding of the neurobiological mechanisms of smoking should not be separated from a multidisciplinary research approach: the aim is to delineate the topography of the determining factors in the various types of smokers, without excluding the considerable individual and genetic variation components.

References

- Corrigall WA. Nicotine self-administration in animals as a dependence model. *Nicotine Tob Res* 1999; 1: 11-20
- De Biasi M. Meccanismi biologici della dipendenza da nicotina. *Tabaccologia* 2006; 1S: 19-23
- Di Chiara G. Role of dopamine in the behavioral actions of nicotine related to addiction. *Eur J Pharmacol* 2000; 393: 295-314
- Heishman SJ, Taylor RC, Henningfield JE. Nicotine and smoking: a review of effects on human performance. *Exp Clin Psychopharmacol* 1994; 2: 345-95
- Merlo Pich E, Pagliusi SR, Tessari M, et al. Common neural substrates for the addictive properties of nictine and cocaine. *Science* 1997; 275: 83-6
- Perkins K. Nicotine self-administration. *Nicotine Tob Res* 1999; 1: S133-S138
- Perry DC, Davila-Garcia MI, Stockmeier CA, et al. Increased nicotinic receptors in brains from smokers: membrane binding and autoradiography studies. *J Pharmacol Exp Ther* 1999; 289: 1545-52
- Stein EA, Pankiewicz J, Harsch HH, et al. Nicotine-induced limbic cortical activation in the human brain: a functional MRI study. *Am J Psychiatry* 1998; 155: 1009-15

14 Behavioral and Psychological Aspects of Smoking

Cristiano Chiamulera [1]

[1] Associate Professor of Pharmacology, Department of Medicine and Public Health, Verona University, Italy

14.1 The Interaction Between Psychological Processes, Behavior, and Environment

The cigarette is cheap, legal, and easy to find; it is used in a context full of stimulating signals (social roles, family patterns, groups, advertising, etc.) with the expectation of pleasant and positive actions, quickly and easily obtained at every breath. In the multidimensionality of smoking, nicotine plays an important role as the best known psychoactive substance (up to now) in cigarette tobacco.

Psychobehavioral effects of tobacco smoking are homologous to those induced by nicotine, and research has shown that many of these have the same neurobiological origin.

Similarly, smoking cessation and withdrawal syndrome have common mechanisms to neuroadaptation (compensation of brain function) due to chronic nicotine

However, dependence on cigarette smoking as a search for gratification and discomfort avoidance requires a definition that includes the inseparable roles of conditioned environmental implications, associated both with pleasure and aversion.

14.2 The Psychobehavioral Processes

The spread of tobacco smoking, with the result that everyone is potentially exposed from birth, contributes to the "normal practice" of the phenomenon. Therefore, in addition to frequent "justifying definitions" (smoking is a habit or a bad habit), this "ordinariness" of smoking gives us a knowledge—based on subjective feelings and social beliefs—of what smoking is and what its peculiarities are. Everybody thinks they know everything, or almost everything, about smoke and smoking.

In the face of the obviously negative individual, social, and cultural consequences deriving from this collective misunderstanding, only the smoker's condition of being lonely with his psychological need to stop smoking (with or without awareness and motivation) remains. It's important to develop a definition of the psychobehavioral processes characterizing the smoker in order to objectify the phenomena and develop a more accurate knowledge of the multicomplexity of smoking. This knowledge, properly translated, has to affect intervention, research, prevention, and collective consciousness.

Robert West and Saul Shiffman [West, 2007] offer us a useful definition of the smoker's complex psychobehavioral process: "A chronic disposition to experience a powerful motivation, to engage in a search for well-being and pleasure, as well as a weakness in inhibiting this activity."

In fact, smoking produces opposing powerful motivational forces. They undermine and weaken the decision to be abstinent, as well as the positive reasons which could lead to smoking cessation.

Motivational processes interfering with the ability to control addictive behavior derive from the interaction among:

- the individual's physiological and psychological vulnerabilities;
- the psychoactive effects of nicotine, and
- the social and physical environment in which the smoker is located.

This vulnerability has been demonstrated to correlate with susceptibility to depression [Karp, 2006], attentional problems, and impulsivity [Rodriguez, 2008] or increased sensitivity to nicotine (the effect of a genetic variation linked to its liver metabolism) [Pomerleau, 1995]. The role of these processes is to leave the smoker in a behavioral mechanism of **habit** (i.e., custom, as an **unconscious automatism**).

The evidence points precisely to this frequent automaticity of smoking a cigarette, when possible, or to the behavior of seeking it if not available, in the presence of signals stimulating the desire [Waters, 2004].

A second type of process regarding the smoker concerns an **appetive dimension**. This looks similar to the hunger for food, even in terms of the subjective descriptions they call forth of an appetitive dimension (e.g., I'm hungry, my mouth is watering, etc.), with the onset of research on the compulsiveness both of cigarettes and of food itself.

These processes are often described as "chemical hunger" in the sense that they are related to plasma levels of nicotine (e.g., the morning after the night of abstinence) [Haberstick, 2007] or eased by replacement therapy to nicotine [Shiffman, 2000]. They are particularly evident in abstinence, where they act as the main cause of weight gain during cessation.

A third type of process is related to an **aversive** type of symptom, or **discomfort**, with mood and affect disorder, irritability, and somatic symptoms. These negative feelings occur with subjective descriptions, with alterations of neurovegetative states (increased skin conductivity, tachycardia, etc.) and with seeking behavior and relapse.

It is well known that this type of process is the most important determinant of relapse in the first days or weeks of abstinence. The smoker, knowing that smoking reduces the stress, the state of malaise, acquires and maintains a carefully regulated behavior of smoking precisely to avoid these symptoms. In general, a state of affective/emotional disorder or a stressful situation can cause relapse even after years of cessation [Shiffman, 2005].

A fourth type of process involves **cognitive functions**. Abstinence from tobacco smoking (and experimental studies also confirm from nicotine) lead to a reduced cognitive performance evident in concentration, attention, and executive functions. The latter are particularly evident as an inability to control impulsiveness and smoking inhibition. This psychological dimension is the subject of recent research as a possible target for intervention in tobacco use, as well as in other types of addiction [Lubman, 2004].

14.3 The Classification of Psychobehavioral Processes in the Diagnostic Criteria of Addiction

Nicotine from cigarette smoking induces a dependence which has been recognized by the World Health Organization [World Health Organization, 1992]. The psychobehavioral processes described for addiction to tobacco smoke are similar to those of other drugs, even if with different modes of interaction and gravity. Therefore, some of the diagnostic criteria are similar to those described for the abuse of other substances, such as the pleasure derived from the use, the abusive or compulsive behavior, and, in the case of cessation, the appearance of withdrawal symptoms (Table XIII) [American Psychiatric Association, 1994].

Craving, also common to other addictions, is a typical subjective phenomenon. Described as a strong uncontrollable desire to smoke, craving has been the subject of various debates about its nature. There is general agreement that craving is the determinant cause of relapse and of smoking cessation failure [O'Brien, 1992]. The seriousness of the problem is that it can also occur after long abstinence periods.

Primary criteria	Additional criteria	Possible symptoms
• Stereotyped model use • Use despite harmful effects • Relapse after withdrawal • Frequent craving to smoke	• Highly regular or compulsive use • Psychoactive effects • Reinforcing behavior	• Tolerance • Physical dependence • Cognitive effects

Table XIII. Criteria of the American Psychiatric Association [American Psychiatric Association, 1994]

14.4 The Environmental Component

The pleasant effects of smoking occur in a stimulating environment and acquire conditioned positive properties which can be very effective in reinforcing cigarette smoking.

Similarly, aversive situations associated with abstinence can lead to relapse.

This strong reaction of smokers to conditioned stimuli, both environmental and interoceptive, is defined as cue reactivity [Niaura, 1988]. Cue reactivity has recently been investigated by means of brain imaging techniques, suggesting specific neuroanatomical and molecular relationships, such as the involvement of the prefrontal cortex areas, the amygdala, and the basal ganglia. These areas are devoted to the integration of memories and emotions and to the environmental information elaboration processes. A recent hypothesis (the "multiple action" model [Chiamulera, 2005]) indicates that the underlying process is an attentional bias to stimuli which are associated with cigarette smoking.

We assume a neuroadaptation in these circuits which sets a different mode of operation, a different homeostasis (**allostasis**) in time.

Repeated associations between smoking and nicotine consumption not only induce gratification in different environmental situations, but also create new pleasant effects and strengthen their memory. Nicotine, and perhaps other mediators, promote the formation of these pleasant memories.

14.5 The Need for a Paradigm Shift

Biological research has shown how the properties of nicotine become relevant for smokers only within a complex context of individual and environmental factors. The environment is deeply rooted and influential within each level of individual memory and the social effects of smoking. This breadth of contextual stimuli associated with neurobiological effects leads to the formation of a the psychobehavioral pattern where the environmental variables intimately interact with the biological ones [Abrams, 1999]. For this reason, categorizations like physical dependence and psychological dependence are too limited to show a view of tobacco complexity corresponding to the knowledge gained in recent years.

It is better to speak of a continuum that, from molecules to behavior, provides insight into the different phenomena and individual aspects characterizing the single smoker.

Psychological, social, and environmental factors have a key role in shifting the balance of motivational pressure far away from smoking and toward cessation.

Nicotine dependence treatment is just one factor, although of fundamental importance, which helps to balance this motivational dynamics [West, 2006].

References

- Abrams DB. Nicotine addiction: paradigms for research in the 21st century. *Nicotine Tob Res* 1999; 1: S211-S215
- American Psychiatric Association. Diagnostic and Statistical Manual of Mental Disorders, 4th edition. Washington, DC: American Psychiatric Association, 1994
- Chiamulera C. Cue reactivity in nicotine and tobacco dependence: a "multipleaction" model of nicotine as a primary reinforcement and as an enhancer of the effects of smoking-associated stimuli. *Brain Res Rev* 2005; 48: 74-97
- Haberstick BC, Timberlake D, Ehringer MA, et al. Genes, time to first cigarette and nicotine dependence in a general population sample of young adults. *Addiction* 2007; 102: 655-65
- Karp I, O'Loughlin J, Hanley J, et al. Risk factors for tobacco dependence in adolescent smokers. *Tob Control* 2006; 15: 199-204
- Lubman DI, Yucel M, Pantelis C. Addiction, a condition of compulsive behavior? Neuroimaging and neuropsychological evidence of inhibitory dysregulation. *Addiction* 2004; 99: 1491-502
- Niaura RS, Rohsenow DJ, Binkoff JA, et al. Relevance of cue reactivity to understanding alcohol and smoking relapse. *J Abnorm Psychol* 1988; 97: 133-52
- O'Brien CP, Childress AR, Ehram R, et al. Conditioning mechanisms in drug dependence. *Clin Neuropharmacol* 1992; 15: 66A-67A
- Pomerleau OF. Individual differences in sensitivity to nicotine: implications for genetic research on nicotine dependence. *Behav Genet* 1995; 25: 161-77
- Rodriguez D, Tercyak KP, Audrain-McGovern J. Effects of inattention and hyperactivity/impulsivity symptoms on development of nicotine dependence from mid adolescence to young adulthood. *J Pediatr Psychol* 2008; 33: 563-75
- Shiffman S, Elash CA, Paton SM, et al. Comparative efficacy of 24-hour and 16-hour transdermal nicotine patches for relief of morning craving. *Addiction* 2000; 95: 1185-95
- Shiffman S. Dynamic influences on smoking relapse process. *J Pers* 2005; 73: 1715-48
- Waters AJ, Shiffman S, Sayette MA, et al. Cue-provoked craving and nicotine replacement therapy in smoking cessation. *J Consult Clin Psychol* 2004; 72: 1136-43
- West R, Shiffman S. Smoking cessation. Abingdon: Health Press, 2007
- West R. Theory of addiction. Oxford: Blackwell, 2006
- World Health Organization. International Classification of Diseases 10th edition. Geneva: WHO, 1992

15 Understanding Personal Motivation. Facing Patient's Resistance With Motivational Interviewing

Fabio Lugoboni [1]

[1] Department of Internal Medicine, Medical Unit for Addictive Disorders, University of Verona, Policlinico GB Rossi, Verona, Italy

15.1 Introduction

Compliance can be defined as "the extent to which patient's behavior (in terms of taking medication, following a diet, modifying habits or attending clinics), coincides with medical or health advice" [Sackett, 1979; McDonald, 2002]. The increased emphasis on prevention in recent years, in fact, has increased the importance of compliance as a factor of success in the treatment of diseases [Johnson, 1992]. If we consider, for example, atherosclerosis, which is the main cause of mortality in developed countries, we will find that almost all risk factors (excluding gender and heredity) can be modified with a medical or behavioral change, but this has not been enough until now to push back atherosclerosis from its dismal track record.

Compliance in the treatment of hypertension has been the most studied; although there are many new appropriate treatments for almost every type of patient, in the U.S. the percentage of good blood pressure control in hypertensive patients does not exceed 27% [Haynes, 2002; Miller, 1997].

It can be even more significant that only 7% of diabetic patients are considered fully adherent to prescribed treatments, and no great differences between the diabetes mellitus (DM) types I and II seem to exist among patients [Evans, 2002]. Of course we have to distinguish (and it is not always easy) noncompliance because of patient resistance from noncompliance because of misinformation or lack of communication, which is also one of the reasons why a patient does not follow certain prescriptions. Even more frustrating are the percentages of patients who accept a medical indication to stop smoking: a simple and explicit call lasting about three minutes is conclusive only in 2% of cases, while a more thorough and detailed intervention (10 minutes), does not exceed a 3% success rate [Raw, 1998].

Patients tend to neglect long-term therapy because drug regimens are often very complicated, expensive, and unnecessary; the disadvantages are often perceived to be stronger than the advantages. The sociodemographic factors such as age, sex, and educational level are not correlated with compliance, which affects all long-term treatments [Stephenson, 1993; Logan, 1996].

The situation is even more worrying because this is often unbeknownst to the physician. It does not predict the subjective clinical impression of successful patient compliance, which is overestimated by about 50% [Boulware, 2001; Mann, 1989]. It was reported that many patients tend to exaggerate their compliance in an attempt to please the doctor, admitting to not taking their medicine in a significant proportion of cases. Another important and complex factor that can make it difficult to identify a lack of compliance is the fact that a patient may be adhering perfectly to certain guidelines and totally refractory to other: for example, some patients attend regular drug therapy but ignore dietary rules, others are compliant at home, but non-compliant when they travel, and others follow the treatment, but not diagnostic tests. Hence, the early detection of low compliance will facilitate the implementation of appropriate corrective actions. Poor compliance entails a large number of hospitalizations, resulting only in the re-introduction of a suspended or never taken therapy, with an important economic and organizational impact for the health care system [Boulware, 2001; Mann, 1989].

Dealing with compliance is not easy: doctors often feel inadequately trained to increase compliance; and it is quite remarkable that so important an aspect of clinical practice is virtually ignored in medical training.

15.2 Improving Compliance

Notwithstanding that the crucial point of compliance is in the doctor-patient relationship, the literature agrees in defining some situations and attitudes useful in improving treatment adherence, which the physician must take into account [Logan, 1996; McDonald, 2002; Haynes, 2002]:

- Set global treatment plans, not only pharmacological treatments (e.g., dietary hypertension).
- Set regimens as simple as possible.
- Negotiate priorities with the patient, and also settle for partial (but effective) agreements.
- Give clear instructions, understandable and weighted to the language of the patient, which take into account the patient's age, sex, habits, and socioeconomic conditions.
- Set regular appointments with tickets as "reminders."
- Advise the patient to keep a therapy journal (particularly important in DM and hypertension).
- Call patients who miss appointments for follow-ups.
- Explain clearly the importance of follow-up.

This allows you to make clear the aims and methods of the treatment that will be used, and has proven more effective than the traditional pattern of access, for example, on compliance in hypertensive subjects; but this may still not be enough.

The patient often does not follow the doctor's advice, not because he does not understand, or because of negligence, but because he is not convinced; and whether we realize it or not, the physician has very limited power to overcome the resistance of the patient.

With the evolving interest in health and the gradually increasing importance of the preventive aspects, the traditional role of the doctor as authority figure has diminished, in favor of a more central and increasingly active role for the patient, which is a healthy process. But to emphasize the role of the preventive means automatically to emphasize communication and awareness on the part of the patient. The establishment of a friendly relationship with the patient, communicative, participatory, never in a hurry, always ready to provide practical advice, is more and more evaluated positively. The objection on the part of physicians or the medical ward, that there is not time to implement effectively a condition of true dialog is, in fact, unfounded, as it produces noncompliance. As we have seen, this most likely leads to acute interventions, direct and indirect expenses, and, last but not least, lower job satisfaction—in general, the perception that "patients now do what they want and use their doctor only when they are really bad."

Of the many variables we have seen, **good communication** seems to be one of the most important. While giving clear, simple, and, above all, written instructions has proved to be essential in improving adherence to proper therapy, the emotional aspect in the doctor-patient relationship is frequently reported as a matter of even greater impact. It is important to emphasize the aspect of emotional empathy, as discussed below, compared to a model impeccably professional but aloof. A study of physicians reported that 100% of their patients had improved on the basis of more adequate blood pressure control, while only 48% of patients felt their success as a therapeutic improvement in quality of life and, in 10% of cases, the situation was perceived as a marked subjective deterioration [Mann, 1989]. But what is good communication?

We communicate not only through verbal language, but also through body and facial expressions and modulating the voice, therefore in a **paraverbal** and **nonverbal** way.

Body communication can take on a truly remarkable relevance in some contexts and it is in health care that what the English called the "healing touch" can express its maximum potential. Sometimes we use it in a spontaneous way, at least when—emotionally—we feel very involved; we're talking about the times when, without saying anything in front of a patient in tears, we lay our hand on his, we stretch to shake his shoulder, we place an arm around his shoulder or hug him. These are things we tend to remember and, above all, that the patient does not forget.

With regard to **duration of speaking**, the doctor interrupts the patient, on average, 20 seconds after he started talking. When the patient stops, it is important to wait at least three seconds, because he often starts speaking again, and the most important things are said at the end. Rarely do uninterrupted patients speak for more than three or four minutes. The following are also useful tips:

- avoid long monologs;
- do not minimize;
- avoid being vague and imprecise;
- encourage and listen to the questions of the patient and family;
- explore and consider the implications of the sexual sphere.

Take account of the emotions. Patients may react very differently to bad news. There may be tears, but also anger, frustration, aggression, anxiety, relief, and gratitude. Not only the cognitive level, but also the physiological one may be involved, with sweating, tachycardia, and altered speech.

If we expect a strong reaction, we'll be less unprepared to handle it; the patient's emotions must be recognized as legitimate ("I understand your anger," "Please take a handkerchief from my table."). Keep talking, giving them an appropriate timeframe ("What makes you suffer more?").

We need to give patients more time to react, because the more we observe their reaction, the better we will be able to intercept it. This is why patients should be listened to quietly and carefully.

This is perhaps the area in which nonverbal communication reaches its maximum successful application.

We should not fear our own emotions, which are also legitimate, nor our silence. Sometimes silence, as we shall see below in cases where the patient is not motivated, is one way to resist the plan of care, but at other times silence is legitimate, because there is nothing to say.

One's physical presence, when perceived as emotional and involved, is the most important support for the patient.

We talked about good communication and simple rules to increase compliance, but all this may break against the "wall" of lack of motivation, whether evident or subtle.

"Give me a fulcrum and I will move the earth." It is just from the feeling of elusive and slippery fugitive intangibility that the low motivation of the patient can weaken even the most sympathetic and caring therapist. In this case, the strategies of motivational interviewing may become very useful.

15.3 Motivational Interviewing

Motivational interviewing (MI) is a kind of relational approach developed in the late 1980s in the English-speaking countries for the treatment of addictions. It is a type of counseling, patient-centred, to address and resolve conflicts and ambivalences in the therapeutic relationship by means of behavioral changes.

After some delay, the work of the main drafters, J. Prochaska and C. Di Clemente [Prochaska, 1991] on the one hand, and W.R. Miller and S. Rollnick [Miller, 2002] on the other, has been translated, and has been widespread in other countries since the mid-1990s. MI is proposed as an alternative to a style of conversation which is very popular in the medical world, defined as "confrontational" [Prochaska, 1998].

In a confrontational dialogue, which tends to identify and dismantle contradictions and patient's resistance, there are often communication blocks that do not solve the problem of compliance, while leaving the therapist with the impression of having done his duty, having outlined by force "what is true and indisputable."

The problem is that the patient, the subject of the change, often takes an attitude that ranges from full affirmation, instinctively trying to please the doctor, to a vague nod, to a more open hostility that increases proportionally with the insistence of the doctor on using guilty tones. All this is often amplified and becomes systematic in the field of addictions, including smoking, of course.

"The pulmonary function tests are increasingly worse. Have you made an appointment with the smoke centre, as we agreed?"

"Doctor, not yet. I tried calling, but I always found the line busy."

"You have to insist! Your wife, who has more time, can call."

"I prefer to call. The problem is that we are so busy this month ..."

"Meanwhile, make an appointment."

"I wouldn't like to make a bad impression by not going and taking the place of someone who is needing help more than I ..."

To try to radically change this approach, which often results in sterile opposition between doctor and noncompliant patient, new MI diagnostic and therapeutic strategies have gradually been refined to induce behavioral change and improve compliance where it is missing or weak.

15.4 MI: The Stages of Change

The difference between "compliant" and "noncompliant" patients, considered as a categorical permanent distinction (like other personality traits such as "meticulous," "punctual," etc.) is too simplistic.

In an MI view, compliance is highly variable over time, and it can be influenced by the therapeutic relationship [Prochaska, 1991]. The changing possibilities vary from the total rejection of every opportunity to the full and unconditional compliance with therapy, in sequential events called "stages of change." As stated earlier, we have already dealt with these matters in the main body of the book, but they are more fully developed and extended here.

The first stage is called **precontemplation**. Patients in this stage are defined as unaware of their condition, not worried, unreasoning, almost incredulous about the objective data provided by the physician, and, above all, not willing to change. The therapist often experiences the unpleasant feeling of being in front of a rubber wall, with the patient rejecting his efforts in an exactly equal and opposite way. In these cases, the doctor often appeals to the patient's family to make him more reasonable, but this usually does not improve compliance. We often encounter patients at this stage when dealing with addiction to nicotine or alcohol, but this is also true for obesity and other harmful ways of life in general.

Although it may seem paradoxical, this stage can last a lifetime.

The next stage is called **contemplation**. It is characterized by the awareness of the pathological condition of the patient, who recognizes the good reasons of the doctor who's proposing a change or treatment.

The strong ambivalence typical of this stage tends to prevent change. The therapist does not experience resistance, but consent, approval, thanks for his zealous efforts—but without the patient deciding to change:

- *"Doctor, I believe you when you say I need to start therapy to quit smoking as soon as possible, but I would expect a little more time to see if I can stop gradually."*
- *"I agree that I have to quit smoking, and I am willing to do so just after the Christmas holidays."*

In this stage we find the majority of noncompliant patients in internal medicine, and in this stage we find most of the nicotine-addicted, if we allow them to be free to express themselves without being burdened by having to make specific commitments. In short, the majority of smokers, when asked if they are going to smoke throughout their life, undoubtedly will tell you no, they will stop sooner or later, especially when sick. In this regard Karl Fagerström says that almost all smokers want to quit smoking, but almost nobody wants to do it now. Patients in a state of strong ambivalence do not deny the disease, the importance of reducing risk factors, and the competence of the doctor; they only defer, seizing every excuse not to change, to suspend the therapy, not to resume it after a temporary cessation, to arbitrarily reduce the dosage. Their false conciliatory approach can easily be misleading. Even this phase of change can last a long time, potentially forever.

Progressing in the wheel of changes, here is the stage of **determination** when patients have finally decided to change. The ambiguities, the excuses, the oppositions are replaced by a clearer therapeutic adherence: they accept the therapy, the proposed treatment plan, the direction to stop smoking, reduce weight, adapt the diet, etc.

The important thing to remember is that, unlike the earlier stages which are potentially long-lasting and offer a slow evolutionary trend, the determination phase is characterized by a very short duration, measurable approximately in weeks. It is therefore crucial that the therapist realizes quickly this change in attitude, in order to begin the proposed change immediately.

The next stage is **action**, marked by full adherence to what is proposed: the patient takes the treatment even in the presence of any side effects; in consultation with the physician, he agrees to hold to a reasonable lifestyle, etc.

Prochaska and Di Clemente argue that this stage does not last more than six months, then gives way to the next, that of **maintaining**—when changes become a lifestyle, fully embedded in the patient's habits [Prochaska, 1998].

At this stage, you can progress to the last stage of change, the one closing the circle—the relapse.

Unfortunately, **relapse** often leads back to a state of precontemplation, basically starting from scratch. This is easily verified in those who start smoking again, forgetting the well-being they've experienced, or regain the weight lost on a diet, and also in those who experience serious side effects to a drug and decide to follow only herbal therapies or unvalidated treatments (pranotherapy, Bach flowers, etc.).

15.5 The Process of Change

Miller, even in the absence of an organic theory, eclectically gathered four lines of thought for MI [Miller, 1993]: the "client-centered" approach by Carl Rogers, the theory of "cognitive dissonance" by Leon Festinger, the theory of "self-perception" by Daryl Bem, the self-efficacy theory by Albert Bandura.

When we come to behaviors that are **maladaptive**, according to our external perspective, but are deeply **adaptive**, from the perspective of the subjective individual history, patients who need a change in these behaviors are in a state of **ambivalence** about that change.

Before analyzing the specific actions to be taken at various stages of change according to MI, it is important to define what the components are that drive a person to change. They are basically three: self-efficacy, inner fracture, and willingness to change.

Self-efficacy is defined as confidence in one's ability to achieve a defined objective. It has to do with self-esteem and with self-love, as observed by several authors [Prochaska, 1991; Bandura, 1977; Prochaska, 1998; Guelfi, 2001; Miller, 2002; Lugoboni, 2008].

We can see self-efficacy as an opening with an upper and a lower margin; and when there is even a virtual opening, it strives for omnipotence, toward the classic:

"I stop when I want!"

With the opening of the wound, the feeling of omnipotence is reduced in favour of a painful perception of not being able to change, soothed by the minimization:

"It won't be too easy, but if I really felt the need, I certainly would quit smoking, without wasting too many words."

The progressive opening of the fracture leads to the ideal level of pressure for change:

"I think I can do it."

The total opening of the "wound" leads to a paralysis of motivation:

"I'll never make it."

This factor can be severely affected by a depressed mood, as depression paralyzes changes and undermines self-esteem; the therapist, whatever his specialty, must be careful in identifying a state of depression, even when the patient tends to minimize it and to correlate it to an organic disease.

In this regard, the use of simple support tools such as self-tests can detect, quantify, and track the depression that may hinder compliance in the realization, often unacknowledged, that every therapeutic effort is actually useless or too late [Bandura, 1977].

The second factor driving change is discrepancy (**inner fracture**), a painful perception of the contradictions between the personal ideal values and the present condition.

The patient comes to the point where he feels it would be intolerable not to change:

"For the good of my family I can no longer neglect myself in this way!"

With the increase of the discrepancy, pain grows exponentially, but, paradoxically, with a paralyzing effect.

It's the painful feeling of having been late for an appointment, without any possibility of a second chance.

"You should stop smoking. You were a sportsman, once upon a time."

"You're right, Doctor, I cannot even take four steps without being out of breath. I know, I suck. Yesterday a friend from the old team barely recognized me. But there is nothing to do. When you've been smoking for a lifetime, therapies are useless. Maybe I should change jobs, but how can I? We are old—this is the bitter, the sad truth. And there is no remedy for this."

The therapist must be careful to reduce the discrepancy within acceptable limits; trying to open it if the patient minimizes, trying instead to reassure and support him if it is too open, never leveraging on guilt. Waiting until the patient hits rock bottom, for instance, by developing a sensible and clear realization that the disease is worsening, is not in itself a driver for change, but often the exact opposite.

The third factor is the **willingness to change**, following the above steps. Each person is at a certain stage of potentially evolutionary change.

15.6 Barriers to Communication

Authors such as Gordon, Miller, and Rollnick [Gordon, 1970; Miller, 1993] analyzed what not to do in the therapeutic dialogue to prevent a lack of compliance becoming a noncompliance. Many of the situations described are quite frequent in medical care and should be avoided because they tend, unconsciously, to undermine the empathic climate that drives the patient to compliance.

What follows is a quick overview of the most common blocks of communication. The examples are attitudes that physicians should avoid.

Giving directives. When you say directly to the patient what he should do:

"With this blood pressure, you should definitely start therapy ..."

Giving ominous warnings. Tips that contain veiled or open threats are disregarded by the patient:

"By quitting smoking you will gain 21 years of life!"

"If you do not quit smoking, you have only a short time to live!"

Making sermons. The doctor faces the problem in a moral way and relies heavily on the sense of guilt:

"Quitting smoking is your duty as a parent of a child with asthma ..."

Blaming, criticizing. Direct blame leads to noncompliance:

"You do not realize that smoking with these blood glucose levels means that your circulation ..."

Shaming. It is often done deliberately to stir the very noncompliant patient (often resulting in an adverse effect):

"Do you realize your stupidity in not taking therapy anymore?"

"But how could you plan to take your therapy in this absurd way?"

Trying to convince with logical arguments. The doctor makes the patient feel inadequate and in error, as if he could not understand the scientific truths held by the therapist. In this way, the patient moves away from compliance:

"You're wrong, and I'll explain where the error is: when you say you only smoke light cigarettes you actually do not know that ..."

Interpreting. This is a very subtle lack of communication; the doctor tries to explain the reason for noncompliance:

"I think I understand why you refuse to stop smoking: you actually are afraid of ..."

Tagging. This occurs when the doctor believes he has perfectly framed the issue:

"I have long experience, you are a typical case of ..."

"Look, according to recent studies, 67% of those who, like you, have ..."

Comparing the denial. The doctor starts from the noncompliance of the patient and, following arguments of cause and effect, nails him in an illogical position—with the paradoxical effect that the patient defends himself increasingly:

"These are the first symptoms. If you do not stop, you will develop smoking-obstructive chronic bronchitis, and subsequently respiratory failure."

"Yes, Doctor, but we all must die someway!"

Playing down in an ironic way. The doctor intends to release the patient's tension by changing the subject rapidly, in an attempt to regain his sympathy. But in fact the patient feels trivialized, not understood in his reasons:

"Enough of diseases! What about the football championship this year?"

In more recent times, Miller and Rollnick, who are probably the leading experts and writers in the field of motivational interviewing, have reworked the problem of communication blocks, preferring to call them "traps." The doctor often falls into these traps, which are really easy to find, raising the patient's resistance, which is the exact opposite of what motivational interviewing proposes [Miller, 2002].

The two authors are keen to stress that it is very easy to trigger these traps and become engaged in a head-on confrontation with the patient, thus destroying a relationship characterized until a few moments before by a good understanding and empathy. In order to avoid these traps, it's very important to know as much as possible about them.

The difference between a spontaneously empathetic conversation and the mastery of motivational interviewing techniques is based on recognizing immediately the extremely slippery ground of communication traps, avoiding or circumventing the resistance that is generated by these blocks. Five types of traps are described by Miller and Rollnick.

The trap of questions

This is really very common among doctors, and may be referred to as the "anamnestic trap"—because it is the hurry to clarify the diagnostic picture with insistent and precise questions, quickly turning the conversation into an interrogation.

It may be objected that thoroughly investigating the condition of the patient is essential for a doctor, and this is true; but, once again, the authors would like to emphasize the style and tone of the interview, which becomes less and less empathetic.

The therapist falls into this trap because his attention is focused on gaining information that could confirm or refute the hypothesis that he has been forming in his head. In a kind of "Rossini crescendo," the succession of increasingly urgent questions requiring very short answers, less and less articulated, continues until the patient becomes passive, emotionally withdrawn, flattened by the rate imposed by the dialogue. In such a complicated context it becomes very difficult to ask really "open" questions and avoid choking the dialogue; let us remember that we are talking about interviewing patients who are not too motivated.

How then to reconcile the need to collect essential information, while avoiding falling into a trap of communication? If you have a medical record with spaces to fill with anamnestic information, you can soften the mechanical nature of the questions with the preface,

"I will ask a few general questions about your life, like your age …" (pause)

The patient may simply respond, "I am 45 years old," and wait for the next question, or he may respond to the implicit invitation of the doctor to provide his medical records in his own way, as if he were asked to describe them briefly:

"I am 45 years old, married with two teenage children. I'm an employee … my job often stresses me and leads me to smoke, much to the chagrin of the rest of the family."

Any additional information, qualifications, address, etc., may be collected and recorded with very short questions when the patient stops his story, as if the doctor had asked a formality, but in reality, was looking forward to letting the patient's story go on:

"You said that your wife and children resent …"

The most common objection to this style of working is the limited availability of time and the need to proceed in order to fill the folder; but in fact the time required is not much more, and all the data will be collected even if not in the written sequential order. Bob Miller suggests not to pose more than three closed questions at time, i.e., those requiring laconic answers ("Yes," "No," "45," "Married," etc.), which do not express the emotional state of the patient. Some closed answers are needed, but building a good conversational atmosphere is essential to arriving more quickly and clearly at the roadblocks, the traps preventing the patient from accepting the recommended treatment, or changing a harmful lifestyle, or undergoing a necessary diagnostic procedure.

On the basis of a personal story it is easier, with brief comments by the doctor, to trigger further reflections and the patient's insights, to discovering, as it were, what cards he is holding ("An employee … my job often stresses me and leads me to smoke, much to the chagrin of the rest of the family."). The patient himself shows us the levers to act upon:

"They criticize you often …"

"Criticize? It's a war! My youngest daughter hides my cigarettes!"

"That's not nice …"

"No, it's not nice at all. But how can I stop smoking? I tried many times, but I always relapsed after a couple of days."

The best way to get the answers is often by not asking questions.

The trap of premature focalization

This occurs when the therapist feels rushed to grasp the fact of the matter; the feeling of perfectly knowing and understanding the context makes him euphoric, confident, prompting him to draw hasty conclusions and sterilizing and cooling the emotional tone of the interview. The patient tends to accept uncritically the diagnostic conclusions of the physician, but often without sharing the solutions he has proposed.

"Yes, yes, I understand. You're describing a typical case of depression, I would say quite serious ..."

"How can I say, Doctor? We're all depressed in our family ..."

"But there are very good therapies!"

"Well, my mother was stuffed with drugs for a lifetime, without any result."

No one ever likes to be tagged, to be defined as "a typical case of ..."—least of all, patients with compliance problems. Some are prompted to accept passively what is proposed, others will raise various types of resistance. When one takes the prescription without conviction, perhaps he will not go to the pharmacy, or will suspend therapy at the first suspicion of an undesired effect—of course without consulting the doctor, and with a sharp tendency to avoid being reviewed.

The trap of the expert

This is very similar and, in some ways, connected to the one above.

Here the patient, instead of experiencing the emotional feeling of finding someone who can help, just feels as if he were a doctor's opportunity to add one more trophy to an already rich collection.

The patient feels like a number, one of many; and the relationship, like the flight of a turkey, crashes shortly after take-off.

There are several situations that can bring down even highly experienced persons in a trap.

Sometimes the social importance of the person sitting in front of us, or the emotional investment we made toward those who sent us the patient, or the hope to succeed where so many colleagues have failed—all those factors can lead us to be too confident.

What really matters is not making whoever stands before us feel like just a "case," but rather as a suffering person; otherwise the relationship will suffer in a negative way.

"I'm glad that you spoke to me about this difficult problem; I recently wrote an article on a very similar case ..."

The trap of the expert raises perhaps less resistance (feeling "a classic case of ..." is probably more irritating than knowing that you are facing the "typical expert ..."), but in this case the adherence to the treatment program tends to be weak and inconsistent, unless there is a strong feeling of "Doctor, save me!"—but this is not exactly the kind of therapeutic relationship we are describing now.

The trap of blaming

Similar to some blocks of communication described by Gordon, the trap of blaming starts with the idea that the therapist has to shake up the patient a little bit, in order to make him desist from nonacceptance or resistance to the doctor's proposal.

It's a very common trap in the world of health care, and it is very often seen in a positive way.

In reality, blame puts the patient in a state of inferiority and unworthiness, pushing him hard to drop out of therapy or, in some less frequent cases, to fierce resistance.

"You're right, Doctor, we are both wasting our time. I will not make fun of you—you undoubtedly have more important cases than mine."

"You are probably right, Doctor, when you tell me that I'm a bad patient, because I'm suspending therapy at the slightest disturbance, but please remember that, at the end of the day, it's my life and there are people who die every year from incorrect treatment ..."

The trap of confrontation/denial

This is triggered when the dialogue is stiff and the patient's resistance tends to be more clear. And the therapist engages in a confrontation dialogue, in which the patient counters each argument for change with an argument for remaining the same. This position, very logical on a rational basis, may cause a strong, further rise of resistance, prompting the patient gradually to defend more and more absurd and impossible positions, in surreal and sometimes incredible scenes. The result is that the patient, pushed into a dead end by the compelling logic of the therapist, defends himself with his nails. At this point, the therapeutic relationship goes to pieces.

"Smoking is a poison to you!"

"I smoke only light cigarettes."

- *"They do not exist anymore—the European Union has banned the term because it's misleading!"*
- *"Instead of dealing with real problems, like pollution, they deal with this nonsense!"*
- *"But with your emphysema, all scientific studies show that nothing is worse than smoking!"*
- *"Yes ... studies which are paid for by the drug companies!"*

Keeping resistance low, trying to avoid communication blocks, is one of the objectives of motivational interviewing. Its "strategies cluster" and techniques can prevent the therapist from falling into the very frequent and insidious traps occurring in the dialogue with unmotivated patients.

15.7 The Five Principles of MI

According to MI, there are five principles to be taken into maximum consideration if you want to orient a patient not adhering to proper behavior.

The first principle is to **express empathy**. Empathy does not mean consent or tolerance of the patient's noncompliance, but acceptance of the person in the changing stage where the person is. This principle can be difficult to accept for the doctor, who tends sometimes to consider the problem in a too apodictic and schematic way. But this nonjudgemental attitude is the best possible compromise between doctor and patient under these conditions.

The second principle is to **avoid argumentation**. It's a common experience that the more discussion arises between doctor and patient, the less the patient is willing to change or accept the proposed treatment. It's as if every doctor's insistence would contribute, paradoxically, to strengthen the patient's irrational defences.

The third principle, **cirvumvent resistance**, starts from the observation that facing resistance frontally tends to strengthen it, so it's a losing strategy. This is also true when, with great patience, the doctor tries to explain the benefits of his therapeutic strategy. Circumventing resistance keeps the patient's defences low and gives him a chance to evolve in the process of change.

The fourth principle, **work on the inner fracture**, means to leverage one of the strongest drivers for change, acting on the contradictions of the patient not at a logical level (which would certainly be easier for the physician, but counterproductive) but emotionally, showing how things are and how they could be.

The last principle, **support self-efficacy**, is accomplished by calling to mind the patient's previous success in health care or in other contexts, making him feel that he can do it.

It's very clear that this principle applies to those who waver regarding the idea of quitting smoking or dieting, but also in changing the patient's stress level toward his work, and tackling challenging surgery or therapy with heavy side effects.

It's obvious that a shaky patient takes advantage of frequent contacts with the physician; in this regard, the effectiveness of telephone contact, as a real event, has been reported; with a minimal loss of time, benefits have occurred in situations where compliance is notoriously as low as smoking cessation [Burke, 2002].

15.8 Creating Motivation: The Basic Skills of MI

If the principles described above can be used to learn the approach to a noncompliant or partially compliant patient, it is possible to learn through basic MI skills a few techniques that may play a positively decisive role in increasing or creating compliance.

Ask open-ended questions

Ask open-ended questions as opposed to closed questions (those that can only be answered with a yes or no or something like that); the open-ended questions tend to stimulate dialogue, a first level situation in case of noncompliance to an adequate antihypertensive therapy [Logan, 1996].

"*What makes you think quitting smoking is impossible?*"

instead of:

"*You absolutely must stop, do you realize that?*"

It might look trivial, but getting used to formulating only open questions, whenever there is resistance in the patient, can offer really unexpected results. Moreover, stimulating dialogue helps to bring the patient's doubts and fears to the surface.

Listen reflectively

Listen reflectively is rephrasing succinctly (in the affirmative, without irony) what the patient has just said, even when it seems frankly laughable, as if it was something we never got to consider, as an interesting point of view. This allows us to refute the erroneous statements of the patient, keeping an empathetic tone, without becoming openly at odds with him, lowering his resistance, and keeping the dialogue open. In its simplest implementation, it means to repeat, to "parrot" what the patient said. In more complex forms, it's to reformulate the statement as if it was preceded by a "you mean that ... ," in the affirmative, not interrogative (which contains an implicit sense of blame) form:

"You mean that quitting smoking is useless."

The patient often tends to rectify what has been reformulated, reopening an otherwise closed dialogue:

"Well, Doctor, I didn't mean that—maybe I explained it in a bad way; but in reality I fear ..."

Support and confirm

This technique is designed to support self-efficacy, which, as we saw, is one of the factors affecting change; it also has a strengthening effect on the relationship with the therapist:

"It's a good thing that you're back, to inform me of this unpleasant side effect that persuaded you to discontinue the drug two weeks ago."

This builds on the positive aspects of the therapeutic relationship rather than on the guilt:

"You should have informed me immediately of the disorder, rather than discontinue the therapy!"

"Never heard that this drug may cause ..."

Knowing how to summarize

This allows you to take stock of the situation, including the ambivalence and contradictions expressed by the patient, replying so calm and reflective, inviting him to participate, correct, and think again.

"So, please correct me if I'm wrong—you would be glad to quit smoking; on the other hand, you do not want to take drugs because ..."

Knowing how to use balance in decision-making

Quite simply, this means to evaluate calmly with the patient the "pros and cons" of noncompliance, of non-change. This is radically different from describing the benefits of the proposed treatment; that way, the patient is encouraged to raise his resistance, with the result that he does not really listen to the good reasons of the therapist. Evaluating the possibility of no change also means accepting and respecting the choices of the patient, asking him to express his fears freely, so that you can reassure and perhaps change him.

"Now, if we decide to forget quitting smoking despite your breathing difficulty, what are you most afraid of in your daily life?"

Elicit self-motivational statements

While the techniques described above are useful to move the patient toward compliance, the ability to evoke in the patient self-motivating statements goes further, trying to trigger the change on the principle that one is most convinced, after all, by his own words.

"Doctor, if you are sure that this drug can really help me, I'm willing to try the therapy."

15.9 Evidence of Effectiveness

MI has been widely applied with success to overcoming dependence on substances (alcohol, tobacco, and illegal drugs), the area in which it was born and developed; a considerable number of studies exists in this area.

At present, controlled studies evaluating MI in general medicine are much lower in number, but their results are very encouraging.

Motivational interviewing seems to be very suitable for the follow-up of chronic diseases, and therefore particularly useful for those working in outpatient and day hospitals [Lugoboni, 2004; Resnicow, 2002; Walitzer, 1999].

15.10 Conclusion

Very briefly, and in the absence of a standard definition, the **strategic components of motivational interviewing** (MI) are [Hettema, 2005]:

- collaborative spirit;
- centering on the customer;
- no judgement;
- building of a trust relationship;
- lowering the resistance;
- increasing the ability to change;
- increasing self-efficacy;
- increasing perceived discrepancy;
- reflective listening; and
- facilitation of change-oriented statements, divided into five additional components [Amrhein, 2003]:
  - changing desire;
  - ability to support change;
  - reasons to change;
  - need to achieve change;
  - commitment to change.

The kinds of strategies gathered in MI represent a good approach to diseases that are very difficult to treat, such as dependence on substances and behavioral disorders; in a few years, MI became the standard approach to overcoming addiction to nicotine in the United Kingdom [Riemsma, 2003].

From this limited scope, MI has been successfully applied in the English-speaking world to other therapeutic contexts such as metabolic disorders, cardiac rehabilitation, treatment of hypertension, and so on.

Understanding the mechanisms that hinder good compliance to therapy and learning some basic techniques can actually improve the quality of doctor-patient dialogue, which, if deficient, is the leading cause of "therapeutic withdrawal" from treatments. Action on compliance has shown significant positive effects in terms of morbidity and mortality. On the other hand, neglecting these aspects can have serious consequences in health care costs because of more frequent hospitalizations and complications. For the doctor who is going to cure tobacco addiction—a chronic disease with a tendency to relapse, and often characterised by strong ambivalence—it is essential to learn how to circumvent the patient's resistance. This skill, with time and experience, will improve adherence to all clinical treatments.

References

- Amrhein PC, Miller WR, Yahne CE. Client commitment language during motivational interviewing predicts durg use outcomes. *J Consult Clin Psychol* 2003; 71: 862-78
- Bandura A. Self efficacy: toward a unifying theory of behavioral change. *Psychol Rev* 1977; 84: 191-215

- Boulware EL, Daumit GL, Frick KD, et al. An evidence-based review of patient-centered behavioral intervention for hypertension. *Am J Prev Med* 2001; 21: 221-32
- Burke BL, Arkowitz H, Dunn C. The efficacy of motivational interviewing. In: Miller WR, Rollnick S. Motivational interviewing: preparing people for change. New York: Guildford Press, 2002; pp. 217-50
- Evans JM, Donnan PT, Morris AD. Adherence to oral hypoglycaemic agents prior to insulin therapy in type 2 diabetes. *Diabet Med* 2002; 19: 685-88
- Gordon T. Parent effectiveness training. New York: Wyden, 1970
- Guelfi GP, Scaglia M, Spiller V. Il colloquio motivazionale nella dipendenza da alcool e droghe. *ADD* 2001; 3: 24-42
- Haynes RB, McDonald HP, Garg AX. Helping patiens follow prescribed treatment. *JAMA* 2002; 288: 2880-3
- Hettema J, Steele J, Miller WR. Motivational interviewing. *Annu Rev Clin Psychol* 2005; 1: 91-111
- Johnson SB. Methodological issues in diabetes research. Measuring adherence. *Diabetes Care* 1992; 15: 1658-67
- Logan AG, Irvine MJ. Ipertensione: compliance ed etichettatura del paziente. In: Swales JD. Textbook of hypertension. Salerno: Momento Medico, 1996
- Lugoboni F, Quaglio G, Mezzelani P, et al. Improving compliance in internal medicine: the motivational discussion. *Ann Ital Med Int* 2004; 19: 155-62
- Mann KV, Putnam RW. Physician perceptions of their role in cardiovascular risk reduction. *Prev Med* 1989; 18: 45-58
- McDonald HP, Garg AX, Haynes RB. Interventions to enhance patient adherence to medication prescriptions. *JAMA* 2002; 288: 2868-79
- Miller NH, Hill MN, Kottke T, et al. The multilevel adherence challenge: reccomandations foe a call to action; a statement for health care professionals. *Circulation* 1997; 95: 1085-90
- Miller WR, Benefield RG, Tonigan JS. Enhancing motivation for change in problem drinking: a controlled comparison of two therapist styles. *J Consult Clin Psychiatry* 1993; 61: 455-61
- Miller WR, Rollnick S. Motivational interviewing. Second Edition. New York-London: The Guilford Press, 2002
- Prochaska JO, Di Clemente CC. Toward a comprehensive, transtheoretical model of change: stages of change and addictive behaviors. Treating addictive behaviors. New York and London: Plenum Press, 1998
- Prochaska JO. Assessing how people change. *Cancer* 1991; 67: 805-7
- Raw M, Mc Neill A, West R. Smoking cessation guidelines for health professionals. *Thorax* 1998; 53: 1-19
- Resnicow K, Dilorio C, Soet JT, et al. Motivational interviewing in health promotion: it sounds like something is changing. *Health Psycol* 2002; 21: 444-51
- Riemsma RP, Pattenden J, Bridle C, et al. Systematic review of the effectiveness of stage based interventions to promote smoking cessation. *Brit Med J* 2003; 326: 1175-81
- Sackett DL. The hypertensive patient: compliance with therapy. *Can Med Assoc J* 1979; 121: 259-61

- Stephenson BJ, Rowe BH, Haynes RB, et al. Is this patient taking the treatment as prescribed? *JAMA* 1993; 269: 2779-81
- Walitzer KS, Dermen KH, Connors GJ. Strategies for preparing clients for treatment. A review. *Behav Modif* 1999; 23: 129-51

16 The Pharmacotherapy of Smoking Cessation: An Update

Massimo Baraldo [1]

[1] Associate Professor of Pharmacology. Department of Experimental and Clinical Medicine, Chair of Pharmacology, School of Medicine, University of Udine, Italy. Anti-Smoking Centre, SOC Institute of Clinical Pharmacology, S. Maria della Misericordia University Hospital, Udine, Italy

16.1 Introduction

The pharmacotherapy of smoking should lose the connotation of "drugs for smoking cessation," portraying them as a "magic potion" that makes you lose the habit of smoking. In fact, using this old concept, aided by the presence in the market of products like the electronic cigarette, menthol cigarettes, and so on, which are difficult to interpret as health care products, the pharmacotherapy of smoking was led into a wrong approach for both the patient who used pharmacotherapy with poor results, and the doctors who simply advised or prescribed without providing any other support to the patient. Misuse of these drugs reduced their effectiveness in both the short and long term. In fact, appropriate therapy must not only be able to help the patient stop smoking, but also to maintain long-term abstinence.

The pharmacotherapy of smoking should be seen like any other form of therapy which aims to cure a disease, in this case, smoking. Smoking is the addiction to tobacco, defined as "a set of behavioral, cognitive, and physiological phenomena developed after repeated use of smoking and [which] typically include a strong desire to smoke, difficulty in controlling its use, the persistence of its use in spite of health outcomes, increased tolerance to nicotine, and the presence of withdrawal symptoms" [American Psychiatric Association, 1994].

In this new millennium, considering the fact that smoking is a major risk factor for morbidity and mortality worldwide, the pharmacological treatment of smoking becomes an indispensable tool for preventing or stopping smoking. After all, considering that 70% of smokers want to quit smoking, there is a clear need for a pharmacotherapy to help them quit.

Although the psychological approach (individual or group counseling) was effective in treating tobacco addiction, the combination of counseling and medication was more effective, as recommended by recent guidelines formulated by Fiore et al. [Fiore, 2008], that classify drugs into:

- first-line drugs [NRT, bupropion (BUP), and varenicline (V)];
- second-line drugs [nortriptyline (NOR), clonidine (CLO)].

The **first-line drugs** have had acknowledgement of their effectiveness and safety, and were approved by the Food and Drug Administration (FDA) for this use. There is also evidence of efficacy for **second-line drugs**, and they are used in various countries; but the FDA has not approved them for this use, and there are concerns about their potential adverse effects [Raupach, 2011].

In this chapter, we will explore mainly the clinical pharmacology of first-line drugs, those being the most frequently used, and we will give brief notes on second-line drugs.

16.2 Nicotine Replacement Therapy

Nicotine acts on the brain cholinergic receptors $\alpha_4\beta_2$, considered the primary mediators of nicotine addiction. These receptors are mainly present in the brain (striatum, cortex, and cerebellum) of smokers compared with nonsmokers, but are also present in many regions of the peripheral nervous system [Staley, 2006]. Animal and human studies are confirming that not only nicotine addiction, but also the aptitude to smoke and the ability to stop smoking have a genetic basis [Mineur, 2008].

The pharmacological actions of nicotine are complex and include effects on both the peripheral and central nervous systems. Nicotine is classified as a stimulant of the autonomic ganglia, although it has a double action, both stimulating and depressive. The receptors activation leads to the release of neurotransmitters, including mainly dopamine, which is able to influence the cognitive functions, as well as neuronal development and the transmission of impulses from the CNS to the peripheral organs. The nicotinic receptor may be **closed, open, or desensitised**, and its state depends greatly on the nicotine concentration present in the synapses. In fact, at low concentrations the receptor is open and responds, while at high concentrations it becomes unresponsive. The desensitisation leads to tolerance [De Biasi, 2006]. The result is a variety of cholinergic and adrenergic effects such as tachycardia or bradycardia, due to stimulation and/or interference with the sympathetic and parasympathetic systems, stimulation of aortic and carotid receptors, release of epinephrine from the adrenal medulla, and stimulation of the chemoreceptor trigger zone.

At the neuromuscular junction, nicotine acts as an agonist. The effects on the gastrointestinal tract are secondary to the effects of parasympathetic stimulation. The effects of nicotine on the cardiovascular system mimic those of sympathetic stimulation: the agonism of nicotinic receptors on adrenal medullary cells that cause the release of epinephrine and norepinephrine. So nicotine raises the systolic and diastolic blood pressure and may increase the inotropic and chronotropic action of the heart. The extent of these reactions is closely correlated with nicotine plasma concentrations.

In conclusion, from a pharmacodynamic point of view, we must remember two concepts [Benowitz, 2008a]:

- the dose-response relationship of nicotine is complex: low doses stimulate systems, high doses depress them; and
- nicotine produces tolerance that develops rapidly.

When the nicotine blood and tissue concentrations drops, the satisfaction levels fall, leading to an increased desire to smoke again and to the appearance of withdrawal symptoms. The activation of the receptor leads to an increase of the flow of sodium, which causes depolarization, whose action is expressed mainly in the activation of two brain centres: the mesolimbic system, in which dopamine is released, affecting gratification and pleasure ("craving" in analogy to other substances of abuse); and the locus coeruleus, which is responsible for the release of catecholamines, leading to an increase of wakefulness and vigilance at the central level.

NRT was the first recognized effective drug therapy safe to treat nicotine withdrawal symptoms and help to stop smoking, available in the market in the mid-1980s. It was a gum, in 1990 joined by other products like inhalers, tablets, nasal sprays and patches. NRT is intended to replace, on specific receptors, the nicotine taken in through cigarettes, reducing the withdrawal symptoms when the person stops smoking. In commercial use there are five types of NRT: chewing gum, inhalers, lozenges, nasal sprays, and transdermal patches, varying in dosage from 2 mg to 21 mg.

A recent Cochrane review, summarizing 123 trials with more than 40,000 participants, which compared treatment with NRT and with a placebo, concluded that all forms of NRT increased the chances of quitting by 50-70%, with a follow-up at six months (Table XIV) [Stead, 2008].

The choice of a product and of the dose is usually based on the number of cigarettes smoked per day and on the free will of the smoker, or the advice of the pharmacist, as these products are sold over the counter. In fact, the rationale of this therapy is based on the **adequate replacement of nicotine** absorbed by cigarette smoking with external nicotine, so as not to display symptoms of nicotine with-

Drug	Efficacy (6 months) [OR (95% CI)]
Transdermal patches	1.81 (1.63-2.02)
Chewing gums	1.66 (1.52-1.81)
Inhalers	2.14 (1.44-3.18)
Lozenges	2.05 (1.62-2.59)
Nasal sprays	2.35 (1.63-3.38)

Table XIV. Effectiveness in the meta-analysis of several NRTs after a median follow-up of six months [Stead, 2008]

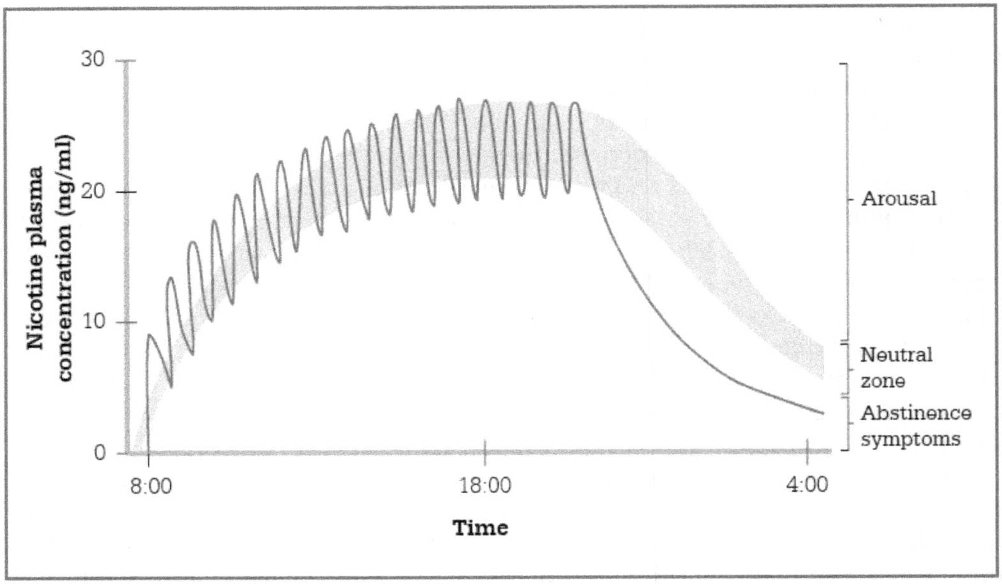

Figure 13. Model of plasma concentrations and daily variation of addiction during a day of cigarette smoking [Hukkanen, 2005; Benowitz, 1992]

drawal; and, once neurochemical and mental balance has been achieved, on a slow and gradual lowering of the dose of nicotine taken, ending eventually in cessation.

Plasma concentrations of nicotine can vary greatly in smokers, primarily depending on two factors: the smoker's characteristics, and those of the tobacco. The **smoker** has some characteristics, such as gender, ethnicity, age, weight, health status, medications, and more, that can affect the nicotine pharmacokinetics, both inter- and intra-individually. The **tobacco** has different amounts of nicotine and can be smoked in different ways; and the amount smoked daily is very variable. All these factors lead to differences in the plasma and brain nicotine concentrations. Consequently, the replacement of plasma nicotine from tobacco smoke with nicotine from NRT cannot always be equivalent, and therefore can lead to a lack of nicotine and obvious signs and symptoms of withdrawal crises.

During a typical day, a smoker reaches plasma concentrations between 10 and 37 ng/ml (Figure 13) [Hukkanen, 2005; Benowitz, 1992].

The highest plasma concentration is achieved in 5-8 min when smoking a cigarette for 5 min, while a transdermal patch of 15 mg/16 hours reaches the peak concentration in 6-9 hours. Plasma concentrations of nicotine in NRT are usually lower than those obtained from tobacco smoke and, at steady state, vary depending on the product: 10-20 ng/ml with transdermal patches, and 5-15 ng/ml with the other products. Even the *ad libitum* use of NRT leads to only 1/3 to 2/3 of the plasma concentrations achieved with cigarette smoking [Hukkanen, 2005]. It follows that, for optimal results from these products, it would be appropriate:

- to define the smoker's nicotine dependence;
- to measure the plasma nicotine and/or cotinine at the steady state of the smoker in order to administer the appropriate dose of NRT; and
- to verify the nicotine and/or cotinine reached after intake of NRT in order to adjust the dosage.

Smokers use nicotine cigarettes to modulate their level of excitation and to check the status of their mood day-to-day. Repetitive exposures to nicotine lead to a neuroadaptation resulting in the development of tolerance to many of the behavioral and cardiovascular effects of the drug. When a person stops smoking and nicotine is reduced, withdrawal symptoms appear. The first cigarette of the morning serves to increase the plasma concentrations of nicotine that fell during the night and causes pleasure (**the first cigarette is always the most appreciated by nicotine-addicted people**), and at the same time increases tolerance. A second cigarette is smoked later, when the smoker feels that there is a regression of tolerance. With the following cigarettes, there is an accumulation of nicotine in the body, evidenced by a slow and gradual increase in plasma concentrations. In the afternoon, a steady state of nicotine plasma concentrations is reached until the last cigarette, which leads to cessation during the night. During this cessation, the concentrations of nicotine go down and there is a resensitization of receptors. Because of the dose-response relationship and tolerance, the majority of smokers

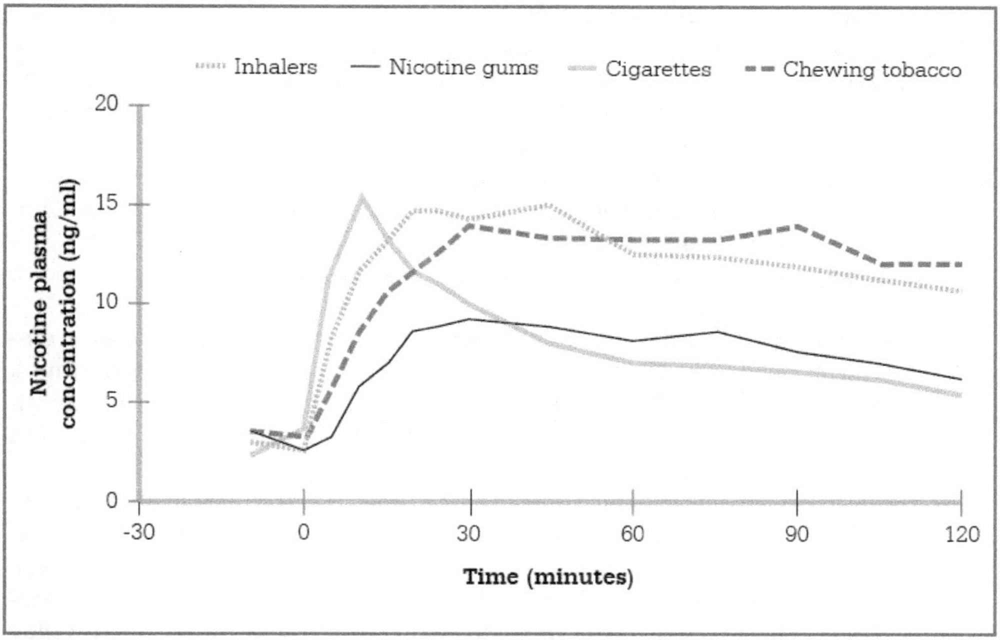

Figure 14. Blood concentrations of nicotine after smoking tobacco, inhalation, chewing tobacco, and chewing gum [Benowitz, 1998]

tend to smoke the same number of cigarettes, at the same time, day after day (especially the strong- and medium-dependent). The smoker adjusts his nicotine level to prevent withdrawal symptoms and maintain a level that produces pleasure and modulates mood, using the same brand of cigarettes, by smoking more or less frequently and more or less intensely, and also by obstructing the entry of the smoke by loosening or tightening his grip on the cigarette [Benowitz, 1999].

Nicotine is a weak base (pKa = 8.0), and absorption through the mucous membranes depends on the pH. After administration, the absorption of nicotine has a variability that depends on the type of formulation [Benowitz, 1992; Hukkanen, 2005]. By chewing gum, absorption through the oral mucosa is easy, but it is slow compared to that obtained by smoking or by the administration by inhalation and/or intranasally, as can be seen in Figure 14.

One study reports that a nicotine lozenge releases 25-27% more nicotine than chewing gum, because the tablet dissolves more completely than synthetic rubber, which releases nicotine depending on the mode of chewing [Shiffman, 2002]. Absorption during 20-30 minutes of chewing varies from 50-90% of the content of the rubber, and the amount absorbed varies widely from person to person. A small amount of nicotine can be absorbed from the GI tract because of its prior metabolism through the liver. The use of acidic foods or beverages such as coffee and cola during, or within 15 min before, the use of chewing gum may reduce the absorption of nicotine, which needs a basic environment [Henningfield, 1990].

After administration by inhalation, nicotine is rapidly absorbed through the mucous membranes of the respiratory tract. Nicotine can be absorbed slowly through the oral mucosa. Less than 5% of an inhaled dose reaches the lower respiratory tract. With intranasal administration, approximately 53% of a dose reach the systemic circulation. After application of the transdermal patch, nicotine is well absorbed through the skin, but the extent of absorption is not known. The peak plasma concentration (C_{max}) since beginning chewing gum can be seen at 15-30 minutes (t_{max}), 15 minutes after inhalation, 4-15 minutes after intranasal administration, and 4-12 hours after application of a transdermal patch. The t_{max} depends on the various products; in Italy, for example, there are patches that need to be used for 12 and 24 hours.

Nicotine is widely distributed in the body and reaches the brain after a single puff, within 7 seconds. Nicotine crosses the placenta and is excreted in milk (mean milk plasma is 2.9:1). The concentration of nicotine in fetal serum and amniotic fluid exceeds that in maternal serum. Measurable amounts were detected in the serum and urine of infants of nursing mothers who smoke.

The plasma concentration of nicotine has a biphasic decline. The majority of nicotine (80%) is metabolized in the liver by oxidation to cotinine and nicotine-l-oxide. This reaction is mediated by cytochrome P450 2A6 (CYP2A6) [Messina, 1997]. Since dependent smokers regulate the amount of smoke in order to adjust the levels of nicotine in their plasma and brain, variations in the activity of CYP2A6 may affect the behavior of the smoker. For example, poor metabolizers of nicotine are associated with a lower consumption of cigarettes, reduced smoking, and reduced intensity of withdrawal symptoms during cessation because they have higher and more stable plasma concentrations of nicotine and do not require frequent compensation for drops in concentration. In addition, these subjects reach higher discontinuation rates in clinical trials. African-American subjects are predominantly poor metabolizers compared to European-Americans. Recent studies suggest that the activity of CYP2A6 may have a clinical utility in determining the type of smoker and the most appropriate treatment [Schnoll, 2009]. For example, the rapid metabolizers could be encouraged to undergo NRT. Instead, poor metabolizers may employ behavioral therapy combined with NRT, but have little benefit from BUP [Ho, 2009; Benowitz, 2008b]. The initial half-life of nicotine is 2-3 minutes and the final is 30-120 minutes, with considerable variation between individuals. Nicotine from a transdermal patch has an elimination half-life of 3-4 hours. Cotinine has a half-life of about 10-40 hours. Nicotine and its metabolites are eliminated via the kidneys, and about 10-20% of nicotine is excreted unchanged in urine.

But who should use these products? All smokers who want to quit smoking can use NRT, with the exception of those for whom this treatment is contraindicated or for which there is insufficient scientific evidence (pregnant women, smokeless tobacco users, light smokers, and adolescents). The guidelines recommend the use of the patch associated with another product *ad libitum*. The choice of the dose and the type of product must be individualized on the basis of previous experience of the patient, his characteristics, his smoking habits, and the presence of oral pathology, dentures, or dermatitis. First, there must be nicotine dependence, which can be determined with Fagerström test. If the smoker has medium-low dependence on nicotine, the percentage of effectiveness is considerably reduced [Hatsukami, 2007; Herrera, 1995; Shiffman, 2002]. Combining two NRT products can be particularly effective in suppressing withdrawal symptoms [Sweeney, 2001; Fagerström, 1994; Bohadana, 2000]. A meta-analysis that compared all therapies with the NRT patch in 86 studies showed improvements in abstinence at six months with patch + gum (OR 1.9, 95% CI 1.3-2.7); patch + BUP (OR 1.3, 95% CI 1.0-1.8) [Fiore, 2008].

The literature shows that women respond less to NRT and thus should be encouraged to use BUP and V [Perkins, 2008].

Recent clinical trials have evaluated the effectiveness of a pretreatment step before quitting smoking, but the results are conflicting and further studies are needed to confirm this hypothesis [Rose, 2009; Etter, 2009].

Because this drug is managed by the smoker, it is often used with even lower doses than recommended and for a shorter period of time [Burns, 2008; Wigger, 2006]. But the customization of therapy (dose and type of product) [Schneider, 2004] and adherence to physician recommendations seem to be crucial for the success of treatment [Shiffman, 2008]. Also key seems to be giving patients the correct information on the mechanisms that underlie nicotine dependence [Raupach, 2010] and the rational use of NRT, and assessing their expectations of success [Vogt, 2008]. Finally, we report in Table XV the guidelines on the clinical use of NRT.

NRT	Dose	Duration	Adverse events
Chewing gum	1-24 cgt/day: 2 mg (up to 24 CW/day) > 25 cgt/day: 4 mg (up to 24 CW/day)	12 weeks	Oral irritation and dyspepsia
Inhaler	6-16 puffs/day	6 months	Irritation of mouth and throat
Tablet	First cgt <30': 4 mg (4-20 tablet/day) First cgt >30': 2 mg (4-20 tablets/day)	Up to 12 weeks	Nausea and heartburn
Nasal spray	8-40 doses/day	3-6 months	Nasal irritation
Patch	21, 14 and 7 mg/24 h 15, 10 and 5 mg/16 h	4 weeks 21 or 15 2 weeks 14 or 10 2 weeks 7 or 5	Skin irritation Insomnia

Table XV. Clinical use of NRT for smoking cessation [Fiore, 2008] (Warning: The information in this table may not be complete. You should see the package insert for each product)

cgt = cigarette; CW =chewing

Nicotine absorbed by pharmaceuticals may have an additive effect with nicotine cigarettes, so patients should be warned about the dangers of continued smoking while taking nicotine outside. Tobacco smoke contains polycyclic aromatic hydrocarbons that can induce hepatic CYP450 microsomal enzymes and increase the metabolism of many drugs. In contrast, smoking cessation can result in increased serum levels and their effects on different drug therapies. Examples of drugs that could be affected are: caffeine, clozapine, oxazepam, olanzapine, pentazocine, phenothiazines, propoxyphene, propranolol, theophylline, tricyclic antidepressants (e.g., imipramine), and warfarin. While in smoking cessation, patients should reduce the dosage of these drugs.

For each type of smoker, with or without concomitant diseases, the risks of replacement therapy should be weighed against the risks of continuing to smoke. The cardiovascular effects of nicotine include peripheral vasoconstriction, tachycardia, and elevated blood pressure. In patients with cardiovascular disease and peripheral vascular disease, the use of patches does not seem to be a greater risk than smoking, provided that the subject does not smoke when using the patch. The transdermal patch has been safely used as an aid to smoking cessation in patients with stabilized heart disease [Joseph, 1996]. However, those with a recent history (within the past two weeks) of unstable angina, myocardial infarction, cardiac surgery, or cardiac arrhythmias should be excluded [Reid, 2010]. Treatment with nicotine should be used with caution in patients with hypertension, pheochromocytoma, insulin-dependent diabetes, vascular disease (e.g., Buerger's disease, Prinzmetal's angina), or thyroid disease resulting in hyperthyroidism or thyrotoxicosis, because it increases blood pressure, heart rate, and blood glucose due to the release of catecholamines induced by nicotine.

Nicotine should be used with caution in patients on sodium restriction to help control blood pressure and/or fluid retention. In subjects who consume both nicotine and BUP there was a higher incidence of emergency treatment for hypertension, and therefore careful monitoring is advisable.

In the case of NRT for the elderly, clinical experience has not identified significant differences compared to younger patients. In general, however, the choice of dose should be cautious, starting with lower doses because of the more frequent presence of hepatic and renal impairment or concomitant disease.

If possible, nicotine should be avoided during pregnancy. Women should be asked to stop smoking through educational and behavioral interventions. The FDA has classified the nicotine released from patches and inhalers in risk category D and nicotine gum in risk category C. However, the information on the use of these products during pregnancy is conflicting.

It is not known whether nicotine can increase fetal heart rate. Spontaneous abortions have been reported in women using NRT, although a real cause and effect relationship has not been recorded. However, since the effects of smoking on foetal and maternal health have been clearly demonstrated (low birth weight, increased risk of miscarriage, and increased perinatal mortality), NRT should be used in evaluating the risk-benefit ratio. NRT should be used with caution in nursing women, because nicotine is distributed into breast milk. However, since NRT leads to lower plasma concentrations from nicotine cigarettes, its use may be considered but should be measured in relation to the risks associated with exposure of the infant at birth to a lower clearance of nicotine.

Other patients at risk are those with peptic ulcers, because the nicotine can delay healing. NRT has not been tested on children and should not be used. Chewing gum is contraindicated in patients with dental disease or in patients with temporomandibular joint disorders. Nicotine is contraindicated in patients with a history of esophagitis, hiatal hernia, or gastroesophageal reflux disease, as these conditions may be exacerbated by the pharmacological effects of nicotine itself. Patients with oral inflammatory diseases could be irritated by chewing gum and lozenges. The transdermal patch may be irritating to patients with certain types of skin diseases, like dermatitis or atopic eczema.

In conclusion, we can say that NRT, although shows good clinical efficacy with reduced side effects and cost, is still ill-used and still has many dark sides. Clinical trials have been conducted primarily on white smokers; teenagers are usually excluded from trials; studies of cigar and pipe smokers are limited; and the subjects who smoked < 10 cigarettes/day were often excluded from drug therapy [Baha, 2010]. Smoking in pregnancy poses serious problems for both mother and foetus, but the trials are lacking [Oncken, 2009]. There are little data on differences in female gender; differences in clinical outcome seem to be related to social inequalities as well [Kotz, 2009].

16.3 Bupropion

There are at least two good reasons to believe that antidepressants can be an effective pharmacotherapy for tobacco use: 1) the symptoms of nicotine withdrawal may cause or precipitate depressive symptoms, and antidepressant drugs can treat them; 2) nicotine can have an antidepressant effect and antidepressants may substitute for nicotine. In addition, some antidepressants may have a specific effect on neuronal components that form the basis of nicotine addiction. BUP and nortriptyline show a clear dependence on the effectiveness of smoking cessation, fluoxetine and venlafaxine have potential effects, and moclobemide and paroxetine do not appear to be effective [Baldessarini, 2001].

BUP is an atypical oral antidepressant, which inhibits the reuptake of norepinephrine and dopamine, with minimal effect on serotonin reuptake [Ascher, 1995; Stahl, 2004]. Furthermore, BUP does not inhibit monoamine oxidase (MAO) and the reuptake of serotonin, and has a moderate anticholinergic activity [Slemmer, 2000]. We do not know the mechanism by which BUP enhances the ability to refrain from smoking, but it may involve a modulation of the mesolimbic dopamine system that would control the craving, and a modulation of the noradrenergic locus coeruleus which would alleviate the symptoms of withdrawal [Arias, 2009; Paterson, 2009].

From a pharmacokinetic point of view [Jefferson, 2005], BUP is rapidly absorbed in the gastrointestinal tract after oral administration, but the bioavailability is < 100% due to the first pass effect [Schroeder, 1983]. The t_{max} is variable depending on the formulation. It is distributed extensively in the body and has a V_{dss} of 19 l/kg. It binds to plasma proteins by 82-88% and easily crosses the blood-brain barrier. Recently it was shown that the human placenta actively regulates the distribution of BUP but not its main metabolite, hydroxy-BUP (OH-BUP) [Hemauer, 2010]. It is metabolized in the liver to three metabolites by pharmacologically active CYP2B6 [Coles, 2008]. The plasma half-life of BUP is about 21 hours; that of the metabolites ranges from 20 to 37 hours and therefore 7-10 days are required to reach steady state [Findlay, 1981]. Approximately 0.5% of BUP is eliminated in the urine in unchanged form.

Enzyme-inducing drugs such as carbamazepine [Ketter, 1995], phenobarbital, phenytoin [Tekle, 1990], rifampicin [Loboz, 2006], and ritonavir may increase metabolism and reduce plasma concentrations of BUP. Conversely, enzyme inhibitors such as ritonavir or ticlopidine [Turpeinen, 2005] can inhibit the metabolism of BUP, increasing plasma concentrations. In addition, bupropion is an inhibitor of CYP2D6 and drugs that are metabolized by this enzyme (beta-blockers, antiarrhythmics, antidepressants) could have their plasma concentrations increased. BUP may cause seizures in a dose-dependent patient [Skowron, 1992]. BUP showed no pharmacokinetic interaction with lamotrigine [Odishaw, 2000].

There were two clinical studies on the pharmacokinetics of BUP in both smokers and nonsmokers which concluded that smoking had no influence on the kinetics of the drug [Stewart, 2001; Hsyu, 1997]. In patients with liver disease, alcoholism, cirrhotic conditions, or left ventricular dysfunction, the half-lives of prolonged exposure to this drug may increase by 1.5-2.5 times. Therefore these patients require a dose adjustment [DeVane, 1990]. In subjects with renal impairment, metabolite concentrations are two to three times higher, and therefore treatment with BUP should be initiated at lower doses in these patients [Worrall, 2004]. Hemodialysis reduces the concentration of BUP and its metabolites by 13%.

BUP is contraindicated in patients with a history of hypersensitivity or severe adverse drug reactions in smokers with psychiatric disorders such as anorexia, bulimia, or bipolar disorder who have taken MAOIs in the last two weeks; with neurological disorders such as epilepsy, or with severe liver disease [Fiore, 2008; Tønnesen, 2007; van Schayck, 2008]. Other factors that may increase the risk of seizures are: alcoholism, head trauma, intracranial tumors or masses, biliary cirrhosis, drug abuse, and concomitant use of antipsychotics, antidepressants, theophylline, tramadol, corticosteroids, opiates, amphetamines, cocaine, appetite suppressants, hypoglycemics, or insulin.

Pharmacokinetic studies in children are limited and have conflicting results, but it seems that development affects the metabolism, leading to a more rapid conversion of BUP in its metabolites [Stewart, 2001; Daviss, 2005]. The safety of BUP has not been evaluated in children or adolescents under 18 years. The clinical need to employ an antidepressant in a child or young adult must be properly weighed against the risk of suicide. Frequent visits and telephone contacts are recommended.

Although pharmacokinetic studies have shown no significant differences between adults and the elderly, the initial and maintenance doses should be reduced in the elderly because of possible reduced liver and renal functions.

BUP is placed in class C by the FDA, and therefore its use during pregnancy is allowed only if the benefits to the mother outweigh the risks to the foetus. BUP should not be used during breastfeeding because the drug reaches the milk and potentially may cause convulsions in the foetus.

In patients with a recent history of myocardial infarction or heart failure, the drug should be used with caution because of demonstrated metabolic depression [Vetter, 2008]. Since BUP can cause hypertension, in some patients, such as hypertensive subjects and those who use NRT at the same time, blood pressure should be monitored.

In the initial phase of therapy with BUP, patients may have reduced tolerance to alcohol and therefore should be warned of possible risks. Those who drive motor vehicles or equipment that requires some attention might have attention deficit and should be warned.

Patients treated with BUP should be observed for the occurrence of neuropsychiatric symptoms such as mood swings, hostility, agitation, depression, suicidal ideation, and suicide attempts [Hurt, 2009]. The most common adverse reactions observed in clinical trials for smoking cessation were headache/migraine, nausea, insomnia, dry mouth, constipation, and agitation. It can be difficult to differentiate these symptoms in a smoker who has stopped smoking and who has withdrawal symptoms. In some cases these symptoms require either the use of anxiolytics or discontinuation of therapy [van Schayck, 2008]. BUP can also cause seizures, but with the dose usually used in smokers, the risk is estimated to be only 1 in 1000 [Hughes, 2007].

BUP has demonstrated a significant dose-related effect [Hurt, 1997]. In 31 trials, abstinence at six months approximately doubled compared with placebo with an OR 1.94 (95% CI 1.72-2.19), a similar result to that obtained with NRT [Hughes, 2007]. If the smoker remains abstinent for seven weeks during therapy with BUP, long-term abstinence is very high. BUP was effective in doubling the cessation rate from smoking compared to placebo, in a similar manner between men and women, and nearly tripling it if in combination with NRT. In fact, the USPHS 2008 guidelines recommend the use of BUP associated with NRT patches [Fiore, 2008; Jorenby, 1999; Scharf, 2004]. As with NRT, appears to be essential, for good efficacy of the drug, a proper patient compliance and confidence in the drug, that should be solicited by correct information provided by the physician [Fucito, 2009]. Although still unconfirmed, it seems that a specific genetic polymorphism may influence response to treatment [David, 2007]. For BUP, it is important to set a date for smoking cessation. Treatment with BUP should start 1-2 weeks before the cessation with 150 mg QD for three days followed by 150 mg BID. The duration of treatment is usually 12 weeks but can continue for up to six months [Fiore, 2008]. BUP has been shown to be cost-effective in smokers with COPD [Van Schayck, 2009]. Combination therapy with BUP + naltrexone appears to be effective in preventing weight gain after smoking cessation in patients who are already overweight [Cahill, 2007]. However, the literature seems to have not yet defined if BUP can be used to prevent weight gain after smoking cessation [Parson, 2009]. In conclusion, BUP alone was more effective than placebo; however, the combination with NRT has given the best results in long-term abstinence. Patients who receive treatment with BUP should be monitored for the onset of neuropsychiatric symptoms, and treatment in this case must be suspended. It is advisable to check for possible pharmacokinetic interactions of concomitant therapy, monitor the possible signs or symptoms, and decrease or increase plasma concentrations of other associated drugs. The ideal patients are those with a history of depression [Fiore, 2008].

16.4 Varenicline

Varenicline (V) is the newest drug approved for the treatment of smoking, and the literature shows that it triples the OR for continuous abstinence at 12 months after initiation of treatment compared with other pharmacological methods [Cahill, 2007].

V binds to the $\alpha_4\beta_2$ subtype of the nicotinic acetylcholine receptor with high affinity and selectivity. It has a dual mechanism of action: a) an **agonist effect** (partial) which results in stimulation of the nicotinic receptors to a lesser extent compared to the nicotine (40-60%); b) an **antagonist effect** which blocks nicotine ability to activate $\alpha_4\beta_2$ receptors and thus stimulate the mesolimbic dopaminergic system, especially in the nucleus accumbens. Similar to drugs of abuse, nicotine increases the release of dopamine in the nucleus accumbens and the prefrontal cortex.

The craving for nicotine is stimulated by low levels of mesolimbic dopamine during periods of abstinence. V is partially effective because it stimulates the $\alpha_4\beta_2$ receptors to produce a modest level of mesolimbic dopamine, causing mild contentment, thus reducing the craving and withdrawal symptoms. This biochemical process compensates for the lack of nicotine that occurs with smoking cessation. Unlike NRT, which by releasing nicotine replaces that of tobacco smoke, obtaining the same clinical effects, V reduces the dynamic effects of nicotine and produces an effect sufficient to alleviate symptoms of craving and withdrawal. V also acts by blocking the receptor sites of nicotine, preventing the effect in the event that the patient continues to smoke. Thus the cigarette smoke does not cause the pleasurable effect the smoker seeks, thereby reducing the desire to smoke.

Treatment should begin one week before the day fixed for the cessation of cigarette smoking and should take at least 12 weeks. During the first week of therapy it will be possible to smoke, and the recommended dose is 0.5 mg once daily for 3 days and 0.5 mg twice daily from 4 to 7 days. The effect of the drug should be to lessen the desire to smoke, and the smoker should arrive at the scheduled day for the complete cessation of smoking with a smaller number of cigarettes smoked. From the day of the cessation, continue with the therapy at full dose (1 mg twice a day) until the end of treatment, which is planned for three months after the initiation of therapy. During the three months of treatment, the smoker must anticipate the loss of daily smoking-related habits e.g., by not drinking coffee after waking, and by reducing or suspending coffee drinking during the day.

V is administered orally and has a nearly complete absorption with high systemic bioavailability (F). It exhibits linear kinetics, reaching C_{max} within 3-4 hours and steady state in about four days. Once absorbed, it is distributed into tissues, including the brain, and has an apparent volume of distribution at steady state (V_{dss}) averaging 415 l. V has low plasma protein binding ($\leq$ 20%) and is independent of age and renal function. There are no controlled studies in pregnant women, although data from animal experiments do not show teratogenic effects at doses up to 50 times the maximum dose used in humans. It is not known if it is excreted in human milk, but it can be found in the milk of animals. 92% of the absorbed dose is excreted unchanged in the urine via glomerular filtration and active tubular secretion; less than 10% is excreted as metabolites. Its mean half-life is 24 hours. There were no statistically significant differences noted in the pharmacokinetics of race, gender, smoking habits, or use of other drugs. In subjects with renal impairment, exposure may be increased between 1.5 and 2.1 times if the creatinine clearance is between 30 and 50 ml/min and < 30 ml/min, respectively. In subjects with hepatic impairment, the kinetics is not altered. There were no statistically significant changes noted during co-administration of digoxin, warfarin, cimetidine, or metformin. It has not been shown to influence the kinetics of BUP and nicotine [Ruiz, 2009].

In phase II and III, V was tested at different doses from 0.25 mg to 2 mg/day vs. placebo resulting in a better and statistically significant abstinence at 12 weeks; with best results obtained at 2 mg twice a day [Nakamura, 2007; Niaura, 2008; Oncken, 2006; Tsai, 2007; Wang, 2009]. At this dose, V vs. BUP was also compared in phase III trials and has achieved better abstinence at 12 weeks with statistically significant differences [Gonzales, 2006; Jorenby, 2006]. It was also compared with abstinence at 12 weeks vs. NRT with results always different and statistically significant [Aubin, 2008]. Data obtained outside of controlled trials found that, as well as NRT and BUP, the **compliance to the treatment** is crucial to achieve continuous abstinence. The interruption of treatment at 2 weeks vs 12 weeks reduces the chances of the patient to remain abstinent more than 90% [Blak, 2010]. Not defining a "**date of cessation**" after the start of treatment corresponds to a significant reduction in the proportion of abstainers in the long term [Hajek, 2009]. V was effective with abstinence at 12 months in subjects with low nicotine dependence as assessed by Fagerström tests, both vs. placebo and vs. BUP [Nides, 2008]. V has shown an acceptable tolerability profile in clinical trials, highlighting among the most frequent side effects nausea, insomnia, and disturbance dreams. These side effects occur during the first week of therapy, may last for two weeks, and decrease thereafter [Parson, 2009; Nides, 2008].

One effect of smoking cessation may be an increase in weight. Although a Cochrane review recently appeared concluding that V can reduce weight gain during treatment, this finding should be interpreted with caution because of missing data for follow-up [Nides, 2008]. Of note among the contraindications and precautions were the following: that V should be used with caution in patients with renal disease, should be used during pregnancy only if potential benefits to the mother outweigh the risks to the foetus, should not be used during breastfeeding, and, because it can cause drowsiness and fatigue, should be used with caution by people who drive cars or use industrial machinery [Ruiz, 2009].

During V treatment, neuropsychic effects were reported, such as changes in behavior, agitation, depression, and suicidal ideation. These adverse reactions develop within days or weeks of starting treatment and may occur both in patients with prior psychiatric disorders and in healthy patients. Therefore patients should be adequately instructed to report any symptoms. In a recent review by Gunnel et al. [Gunnel, 2009], which evaluated 80,660 patients treated with NRT, BUP, and V, out of whom 3.7% had had previous consultations for mental illness, the relative risk of suicidal thoughts was higher for V compared to BUP and NRT.

In a multicenter, randomized, double-blind, placebo-controlled trial to test the safety and efficacy of V in smoking cessation among 714 smokers aged 35-75 years

(≥ 10 cigarettes/day) who had a stable and documented cerebrovascular disease, cardiovascular disease (excluding hypertension alone), or peripheral vascular disease diagnosed > 2 months before screening, V was effective at 12 and 52 weeks [Rigotti, 2010]. However, in a recent review, Singh et al. have shown that in these patients V was associated with a significantly increased risk of serious cardiovascular adverse events compared with placebo (V group 1.06% vs. placebo group 0.82%, OR 1.72, 95% CI 9.1-2.71) [Singh, 2011]. However, according to other authors, the increase of 72% risk of developing adverse cardiovascular effects should be scaled based on the rarity of these events in the V group and placebo group (1.06% vs. 0.82%), with a difference of only 0.24% [Hays, 2011]. Furthermore, according to other authors, the statistical method used by Singh et al. would not be the most appropriate. Re-evaluating the data using the Mantel-Haenszel method, an OR 1.56, 95% CI 0.99-2.44 would have been achieved, smaller and not significantly different from the placebo [Tagagi, 2011]. Therefore, **the small risk of cardiovascular events associated with the use of V in patients with cardiovascular disease is negligible compared to the enormous benefit of reducing morbidity and mortality, which is achieved by stopping smoking**, as confirmed by the European Medicines Agency.

The clinical trials performed so far have yielded encouraging results, but clinical experience is still insufficient to make a definitive judgement on the effectiveness of this new drug. For the moment we can say that we have a new molecule which increases the availability of drugs for the treatment of smoking. Of course, as reported by Klesges et al. in a recent editorial, V is not the panacea for smoking cessation and now will require a much broader study phase to confirm the results [Tonstad, 2006; Klesges, 2006].

In conclusion, **V seems to be currently the most effective drug for the treatment of smoking**. The drug can be taken orally, and has no contraindications or interactions with other drugs. The most common side effects are often dose- and time-related. Attention must be paid in the case of psychiatric patients with previous suicidal episodes. Given the well-known high incidence of smoking-related diseases and mortality, the drug should always be used with a risk-benefit approach rather than risk aversion.

16.5 Second-line Drugs

The second-line drugs for smoking cessation do not currently have this indication and therefore cannot be used for this purpose. According to the guidelines [Fiore, 2008], they should be used in patients who cannot take the first-line drugs because of contraindications, or when the latter have not resulted in good outcomes. They will be briefly mentioned here for completeness of information.

Nortriptyline

Nortriptyline (NOR) is a tricyclic antidepressant that doubles the chances of smokers abstaining from smoking after six months compared to placebo [Hughes, 2007]. The efficacy of nortriptyline is independent of its antidepressant effect and acts by inhibiting the reuptake of serotonin and norepinephrine. It also seems to act by a weak nicotinic receptor antagonism [Hughes, 2005].

Nortriptyline as a single therapy for smoking cessation was better than placebo (n 975, OR 2.34, 95% CI 1.61-3.41), but it has an effect similar to NRT. The association with NRT has been shown to increase smoking cessation without impacting significantly on withdrawal symptoms [Prochaska, 2004]. Comparing BUP with nortriptyline [Haggsträm, 2006; Wagena, 2005], trials have shown better performance than BUP, but without statistically significant differences.

Adverse reactions are those of tricyclic antidepressants related to the blockade of muscarinic cholinergic receptors (dry mouth, blurred vision, constipation, and urinary retention), histamine H_1 receptors (sedation, drowsiness, weight gain), and adrenergic α_1 receptors (orthostatic hypotension) [Fiore, 2008]. Because of the cardiotoxic effects, nortriptyline should be used with extreme caution in patients with cardiovascular disease [Fiore, 2008].

Treatment should be started 10-28 days before the day of smoking cessation. The initial dose should be 25 mg/day, gradually increasing the dose up to 75-100 mg/day for a treatment period of about 12 weeks.

Clonidine

Clonidine is an α_2 noradrenergic agonist and has been shown to reduce withdrawal symptoms caused by opiates and alcohol [Henningfield, 2005]. Treatment with clonidine should start about three days before the day of smoking cessation. The usual starting dose is 0.10 mg twice a day orally or 0.10 mg/day transdermally, increasing 0.10 mg/day per week for a period ranging from three to 10 weeks.

A review of the literature shows that treatment with clonidine is associated with increased cessation after 12 weeks, which is approximately double compared to placebo (OR 1.89, 95% CI 1.30-2.74) [Gourlay, 2000]. Some studies suggest that clonidine is more effective in women than in men [Hilleman, 1993].

The most reported adverse reactions were dry mouth (40%), somnolence (33%), dizziness (16%), sedation (10%), and constipation (10%); but the most dangerous were allergic reactions, bradycardia, and changes in blood pressure that limit its use [Ebbert, 2010].

Drugs under sperimentation: Vaccines

Interest is growing in the possibility of the use of vaccines to treat tobacco addiction [Leader, 2010]. Although beyond the scope of this chapter, because the vaccines are still being tested and are not yet reported by the guidelines, we believe it will be useful to give a brief update.

Nicotinic vaccination [Cerny, 2009] relies on the fact that a molecule of nicotine, suitably treated, can bind with the antibody in the periphery, and therefore the complex nicotine-antibody, because of its size, cannot cross the BEE. This therapy does not require the daily use of drugs, only a periodic vaccination to maintain high antibody titer. Vaccination can be used for the prevention of relapses by blocking the rewarding effect of occasional smoking, in the smoker who decides to quit, or for primary prevention in adolescents [Pentel, 2002].

Preclinical trials have been performed already, in which it was shown that the complex nicotine-antibody significantly changes the pharmacokinetics of nicotine [Hieda, 1997; Pentel, 2000] and can interfere with self-administration [LeSage, 2006; Lindblom, 2002]. Clinical phase I and II trials have not been able to replicate the encouraging results obtained with animal experiments [Hatsukami, 2005; Maurer, 2005; Wagena, 2008; Hatsukami, 2011]. Further studies are needed to clarify the real role of this therapeutic approach.

16.6 Conclusion

In conclusion, drug therapy associated with counseling should be offered to all smokers who want to quit smoking. Each drug of first or second choice has shown evidence of efficacy when used as monotherapy compared to placebo [Fiore, 2008]. However, even with these drugs, only half of the smokers quit smoking after three months and more than two thirds resume smoking after one year. Moreover, heavy smokers often report experiences of craving and withdrawal symptoms even at recommended doses. Trials and clinical experience have shown that the combination of multiple drug therapies can reduce these effects and increase abstinence from smoking. The combination of drugs with the same mechanism of action but different pharmaceutical formulation (NRT), or with different mechanisms of action (NRT + BUP, V + BUP, nortriptyline + NRT, V + NRT), may result in therapeutic synergism [Ebbert, 2010].

The choice of drug therapy should be addressed to one drug or a combination of two drugs. The active substance and/or the type of pharmaceutical product should be chosen on the basis of the following factors [Fiore, 2008; Cofta-Woerpel, 2006]:

- clinical familiarity with the drug;
- the availability of prescription and cost-benefit evaluation; and
- patient characteristics, such as type of smoking history and smoking status, product preferences, previous experiences, and contraindications for existing illnesses.

References

- American Psychiatric Association. Diagnostic and Statistical Manual of Mental Disorder: DSM-IV, 4th edition. Washington, DC: American Psychiatric Press, 1994
- Arias HR. Is the inhibition of nicotinic acetylcholine receptors by bupropion involved in its clinical actions? *Int J Biochem Cell Biol* 2009; 41: 2098-108
- Ascher JA, Cole JO, Colin JN, et al. Bupropion: a review of its mechanism of antidepressant activity. *J Clin Psychiatry* 1995; 56: 395-401
- Aubin HJ, Bobak A, Britton JR, et al. Varenicline versus transdermal nicotine patch for smoking cessation: results from a randomized open-label trial. *Thorax* 2008; 63: 717-24
- Baha MY, Le Faou AL. Smoking cessation intervention offered to French adult light smoker: a heterogeneous population with specificic needs. *Eur Addict Res* 2010; 16: 162-9
- Baldessarini RJ. Drugs and the treatment of psychiatric disorders: depression and ansiety disorders. In: Hardman JC, Limbird LE (eds). Goodman and Gilman's the pharmacological basis of theraputics. New York, NY: McGraw-Hill, 2001; pp. 447-83
- Benowitz NL, Jacob P 3rd. Pharmacokinetics and metabolism of nicotine and related alkaloids. In: Arneric SP, Brioni JD (eds). Neuronal nicotinic receptors: pharmacology and therapeutic opportunities. New York, NY: Wiley-Liss, 1998; pp. 211-*34*
- Benowitz NL. Cigarette smoking and nicotine addiction. *Med Clin North Am* 1992; 76: 415-37
- Benowitz NL. Clinical pharmacology of nicotine: implications for understanding, preventing and treating tobacco addiction. *Clin Pharmacol Ther* 2008a; 83: 531-41
- Benowitz NL. Genetic influence in the variation in renal clearance of nicotine and cotinine *Clin Pharmacol Ther* 2008b; 84: 243-7
- Benowitz NL. Nicotine addiction. *Prim Care* 1999; 26: 611-31
- Blak BT, Wilson K, Metcalfe M, et al. Evaluation of varenicline as an aid to smoking cessation in UK general practice: a THIN database study. *Curr Med Res Opin* 2010; 26: 861-70
- Bohadana A, Nilsson F, Rasmussen T, et al. Nicotine inhaler and nicotine patch as a combination therapy for smoking cessation: a randomized, double-blind, placebo controlled trial. *Arch Intern Med* 2000; 160: 3128-34
- Burns EK, Levison AH. Discontinuation of nicotine replacement therapy among smoking-cessation attempters. *Am J Prev Med* 2008; 34: 212-5
- Cahill K, Stead LF, Lancaster T. Nicotine receptor partial agonists for smoking cessation. *Cochrane Database Syst Rev* 2007; 24: CD006103
- Cerny EH, Cerny T. Vaccines against nicotine. *Hum Vaccin* 2009; 5: 200-5
- Cofta-Woerpel L, Wright KL, Wetter DW. Smoking cessation 1: pharmacological treatments. *Behav Med* 2006; 32: 47-56
- Coles R, Kharasch ED. Stereoselective metabolism of bupropion by cytochrome P4502B6 (CYP2B6) and human liver microsomes. *Pharm Res* 2008; 25: 1405-11
- David SP, Brown RA, Papandonatos GD, et al. Pharmacogentic clinical trial of sustained-release bupropion for smoking cessation. *Nicotine Tob Res* 2007; 9: 821-33

- Daviss WB, Perel JM, Rudolph GR, et al. Steady-state pharmacokinetics of bupropion SR in juvenile patients. *J Am Acad Child Adolesc Psychiatry* 2005; 44: 349-57
- De Biasi M. The biology of nicotine addiction. *Tobaccology* 2006; 1S: 19-23
- DeVane CL, Laizure SC, Stewart JT, et al. Disposition of bupropion in healthy volunteers and subjects with alcoholic liver disease. *J Clin Psychopharmacol* 1990; 10: 328-32
- Ebbert JO, Hays JT, Hurt RD. Combination pharmacotherapy for stopping smoking: what advantages does it offer? *Drugs* 2010; 70: 643-50
- Etter JF, Huguelet P, Perneger TV, et al. Nicotine gum treatment before smoking cessation: a randomized trial. *Arch Intern Med* 2009; 169: 1028-34
- Fagerström KO. Combined use of nicotine replacement products. *Health Values* 1994; 18: 15-20
- Findlay JW, Van Wyck Fleet J, Smith PG, et al. Pharmacokinetics of bupropion, a novel antidepressant agent, following oral administration to healthy subjects. *Eur J Clin Pharmacol* 1981; 21: 127-35
- Fiore MC, Jaen CR, Baker WC, et al. Treating Tobacco use and dependence: 2008 update. Clinical practice guideline. Rockville, MDUS: Department of Health and Human Services, Public Health Service, 2008
- Fucito LM, Toll BA, Salovey P, et al. Beliefs and attitudes about bupropion: implications for medication adherence and smoking cessation treatment. *Psychol Addict Behav* 2009; 23: 373-9
- Gonzales D, Rennard SI, Nides M, et al. Varenicline, an $\alpha_4\beta_2$ nicotinic acetylcholine receptor partial agonist, vs sustained-release bupropion and placebo for smoking cessation: a randomized controlled trial. *JAMA* 2006; 296: 47-55
- Gourlay SG, Stead LF, Benowitz NL. Clonidine for smoking cessation. *Cochrane Database Syst Rev* 2000; 2: CD000058
- Gunnell D. Varenicline and suicidal behavior: a cohort study based on data from the general practice research database. *BMJ* 2009; 339: b3805
- Haggsträm FM, Chatkin JM, Sussenbach-Vaz E, et al. A controller trial of nortriptyline, sustained-release bupropion and placebo for smoking cessation: preliminary results. *Pulm Pharmacol Ther* 2006; 19: 205-9
- Hajek P, Tønnesen P, Arteaga C, et al. Varenicline in prevention of relapse to smoking: effect of quit pattern on response to extended treatment. *Addiction* 2009; 104: 1597-602
- Hatsukami D, Money M, Murphy S, et al. Effects of high dose transdermal nicotine replacement in cigarette smokers. *Pharmacol Biochem Behav* 2007; 86: 132-9
- Hatsukami DK, Jorenby DE, Gonzales D, et al. Immunogenicity and smoking-cessation outcomes for a novel nicotine immunotherapeutic. *Clin Pharmacol Ther* 2011; 89: 392-9
- Hatsukami DK, Rennard S, Jorenby D, et al. Safety and immunogeni city of a nicotine conjugate vaccine in current smokers. *Clin Pharmacol Ther* 2005; 78: 456-67
- Hays JT. Varenicline for smoking cessation: is it a heartbreaker? *CMAJ* 2011; 183: 1346-7
- Hemauer SJ, Patrikeeva SL, Wang X, et al. Role of transporter-mediated efflux in the placental biodisposition of bupropion and its metabolite, OH-bupropion. *Biochem Pharmacol* 2010; 80: 1080-6

- Henningfield JE, Fant RV, Buchhalter AR, et al. Pharmacotherapy for nicotine dependance. *Cancer J Clin* 2005; 55: 281-99
- Henningfield JE, Radzius A, Cooper TM, et al. Drinking coffee and carbonated beverages blocks absorption of nicotine from nicotine polacrilex gum. *JAMA* 1990; 264: 1560-4
- Herrera N, Franco R, Herrera L, et al. Nicotine gum, 2 and 4 mg, for nicotine dependence. A double-blind placebo-controlled trial within a behavior modification support program. *Chest* 1995; 108: 447-51
- Hieda Y, Keyler DE, Vandevoort JT, et al. Active immunization alters the plasma nicotine concentrations in rats. *J Pharmacol Exper Ther* 1997; 283: 1076-81
- Hilleman DE, Mohiuddin SM, Delcore MG, et al. Randomized, controlled trial of transdermal clonidine for smoking cessation. *Ann Pharmacother* 1993; 27: 1025-8
- Ho MK, Mwenifumbo JC, Al Koudsi N, et al. Association of nicotine metabolite ratio and CyP2A6 genotype with smoking cessation treatment in African-American light smokers. *Clin Pharmacol Ther* 2009; 85: 635-43
- Hsyu PH, Singh A, Giargiari TD, et al. Pharmacokinetics of bupropione and its metabolites in cigarette smokers versus nonsmokers. *J Clin Pharmacol* 1997; 37: 737-43
- Hughes J, Stead L, Lancaster T. Antidepressant for smoking cessation. *Cochrane Database Syst Rev* 2007; (1): CD000031
- Hughes Jr, Stead LF, Lancaster T, et al. Nortriptyline for smoking cessation: a review. *Nicotine Tob Res* 2005; 7: 491-9
- Hukkanen J, Jacob P, Benowitz NL. Metabolism and disposition kinetics of nicotine. *Pharmacol Rev* 2005; 57: 79-115
- Hurt R, Sachs D, Glover E, et al. A comparison of susteined-release bupropion and placebo for smoking cessation. *N Engl J Med* 1997; 337: 1195-202
- Hurt RD, Ebbert JO, Hays JT, et al. Treating tobacco dependence in a medical setting. CA *Cancer J Clin* 2009; 59: 314-26
- Jefferson JW, Pradko JF, Muir KT. Bupropion for major depressive disorder: pharmacokinetic and formulation considerations. *Clin Ther* 2005; 27: 1685-95
- Jorenby DE, Hays JT, Rigotti NA, et al. Efficacy of varenicline, an $\alpha_4\beta_2$ nicotinic acetylcholine receptor partial agonist, vs. placebo or sustained-release bupropion for smoking cessation: a randomized controlled trial. *JAMA* 2006; 296: 56-63
- Jorenby DE, Leischow Sj, Nides MA, et al. A controlled trial of sustained-release bupropion, a nicotine patch, or both for smoking cessation. *N Engl J Med* 1999; 340: 685-91
- Joseph AM, Norman SM, Ferry LH, et al. The safety of transdermal nicotine as an aid to smoking cessation in patients with cardiac disease. *N Engl J Med* 1996; 335: 1792-8
- Ketter TA, Jenkins JB, Schroeder DH, et al. Carbamazepine but not valproate induces bupropion metabolism. *J Clin Psychopharmacol* 1995; 15: 327-33
- Klesges RC, Johnson KC, Somes G. Varenicline for smoking cessation. Definite promise, but no panacea. *JAMA* 2006; 296: 94-5
- Kotz D, West R. Explaining the social gradient in smoking cessation: it's not in the trying, but in the succeding. *Tob Control* 2009; 18: 43-6

- Leader AE, Lerman C, Cappella JN. Nicotine vaccines: will smokers take a shot at quitting? *Nicotine Tob Res* 2010; 12: 390-7
- LeSage mg, Keyler DE, Hieda Y, et al. Effects of a nicotine conjugate vaccine on the acquisition and maintenance of nicotine self-administration in rats. *Psycopharmacology* 2006; 184: 409-16
- Lindblom N, de Villiers SH, Kalayanov G, et al. Active immunization against nicotine prevents reinstatement of nicotine-seeking behavior in rats. *Respiration* 2002; 69: 254-60
- Loboz KK, Gross AS, Williams KM, et al. Cytochrome P450 2B6 activity as measured by bupropion hydroxylation: effect of induction by rifampin and ethnicity. *Clin Pharmacol Ther* 2006; 80: 75-84
- Maurer P, Jennings GT, Willers J, et al. A therapeutic vaccine for nicotine dependence: preclinical efficacy ad phase I safety and immunogenicity. *Eur J Immunol* 2005; 35: 2031-40
- Messina ES, Tyndale RF, Sellers EM. A major role for CyP2A6 in nicotine C-oxidation by human liver microsomes. *J Pharmacol Exp Ther* 1997; 282: 1608-14
- Mineur YS, Picciotto MR. Genetics of nicotine acetylcholine receptors: relevance to nicotine addiction. *Biochem Pharmacol* 2008; 75: 323-33
- Nakamura M, Oshima A, Fujimoto Y, et al. Efficacy and tollerability of varenicline, an $\alpha_4\beta_2$ nicotinic acetylcholine receptor partial agonist, in a 12-week, randomized, placebo controlled, dose-response study with 40-week follow-up for smoking cessation in Japanese smokers. *Clin Ther* 2007; 29: 1040-56
- Niaura R, Hays JT, Jorenby DE, et al. The efficacy and safety of vareniclina for smoking cessation using a flexible dosing strategy in adult smokers: a randomized controlled trial. *Curr Med Res Opin* 2008; 24: 1931-41
- Nides M, Glover ED, Reus VI, et al. Varenicline versus bupropion SR or placebo for smoking cessation: a pooled analysis. *Am J Health Behav* 2008; 32: 664-75
- Odishaw J, Chen C. Effects of steady-state bupropion on the pharmacokinetics of lamotrigine in healthy subjects. *Pharmacotherapy* 2000; 20: 1448-53
- Oncken C, Gonzales D, Nides M, et al. Efficacy and safety of the novel selective nicotinic acetylcholine receptor partial agonist, varenicline, for smoking cessation. *Arch Intern Med* 2006; 166: 1571-7
- Oncken CA, Kranzler HR. What do we know about the role of pharmacotherapy for smoking cessation before or during pregnancy. *Nicotine Tob Res* 2009; 11: 1265-73
- Parson AC, Shraim M, Inglis J, et al. Intervention for preventing weight gain after smoking cessation. *Cochrane Database Sys Rev* 2009; (1): CD006219
- Paterson NE. Behavioral and pharmacological mechanisms of bupropion's anti-smoking effects: recent preclinical and clinical insights. *Eur J Pharmacol* 2009; 603: 1-11
- Pentel P, Malin D. A vaccine for nicotine dependence: targeting the drug rather than the brain. *Respiration* 2002; 69: 193-7
- Pentel PR, Malin DH, Ennifar S, et al. A nicotine conjugate vaccine reduces nicotine distribution to brain and attenuates its behavioral and cardiovascular effects in rats. *Pharmacol Biochem Behav* 2000; 65: 191-8

- Perkins KA, Scott J. Sex differences in long-term smoking cessation rates due to nicotine patch. *Nicotine Tob Res* 2008; 10: 1245-50
- Prochaska AV, Kick S, Steinbrunn C, et al. A randomized trial of nortriptyline combined with transdermal nicotine for smoking cessation. *Arch Intern Med* 2004; 164: 2229-33
- Raupach T, Shahab L, Elmer S, et al. Increasing the use of nicotine replacement therapy by a simple intervention: an exploratory trial. *Subst Use Misuse* 2010; 45: 403-13
- Raupach T, van Schayck CP. Pharmacotherapy for smoking cessation. Current advances and research topics. *CNS Drugs* 2011; 25: 371-82
- Reid RD, Mullen KA, Slovinec D'Angelo ME, et al. Smoking cessation for hospitalized smokers: an evaluation of the "Ottawa Model". *Nicotine Tob Res* 2010; 12: 11-8
- Rigotti NA, Pipe AL, Benowitz NL, et al. Efficacy and safety of varenicline for smoking cessation in patients with cardiovascular disease: a randomized trial. *Circulation* 2010; 121: 221-9
- Rose JE, Herskovic JE, Behm FM, et al. Precessation treatment with nicotine patch significantly increases abstinence rates relative to conventional treatment. *Nicotine Tob Res* 2009; 11: 1067-75
- Ruiz CJ, Berlin I, Hering T. Varenicline. A novel pharmacotherapy for smoking cessation. *Drugs* 2009; 69: 1319-38
- Scharf D. Are there gender differences in smoking cessation, with and without bupropion? Pooled- and meta-analyses of clinical trials of bupropione SR. *Addiction* 2004; 99: 1462-9
- Schneider NG, Olmstead RE, Nides M, et al. Comparative testing of 5 nicotine system: initial use and preferences. *Am J Health Behav* 2004; 28: 72-86
- Schnoll RA, Patterson F, Wileyto Et, et al. Nicotin metabolic rate predicts successful smoking cessation with transdermal nicotine: a validation study. *Pharmacol Biochem Behav* 2009; 92: 6-11
- Schroeder DH. Metabolism and kinetics of bupropion. *J Clin Psychiatry* 1983; 44: 79-81
- Shiffman S, Dresler CM, Hajek P, et al. Efficacy of a nicotine lozenge for smoking cessation. *Arch Intern Med* 2002; 162: 1267-76
- Shiffman S, Sweeney CT, Ferguson SG, et al. Relationship between adherence to daily nicotine patch use and treatment efficacy: secondary analysis of a 10-week randomized, double-blind, placebo-controlled clinical trial simulating over-the counter use in adult smokers. *Clin Ther* 2008; 30: 1852-8
- Singh S, Loke YK, Spangler JG, et al. Risk of serious adverse cardiovascular events associated with varenicline: a systematic review and meta-analysis. *CMAJ* 2011; 183: 1359-66
- Skowron DM, Stimmel GL. Antidepressants and the risk of seizures. *Pharmacotherapy* 1992; 12: 18-22
- Slemmer JE, Martin BR, Damaj MI. Bupropion is a nicotinic antagonist. *J Pharmacoll Exp Ther* 2000; 295: 321-7
- Stahl SM, Pradko JF, Haight BR, et al. A review of the neuropharmacology of bupropion, a dual norepinephrine and dopamine reuptake inhibitor. *Prim Care Companion J Clin Psychiatry* 2004; 6: 159-66

- Staley JK, Krishnan-Sarin S, Cosgrove KP, et al. Human tobacco smokers in early abstinence have higher levels of α4β2 nicotinic acethylcholine receptors than nonsmokers. *J Neurosci* 2006; 26: 8707-14
- Stead L, Perera R, Bullen C, et al. Nicotine replacement therapy for smoking cessation. *Cochrane Database Sys Rev* 2008; (1): CD000146
- Stewart JJ, Berkel H J, Parish RC, et al. Single-dose pharmacokinetics of bupropion in adolescents: Effects of smoking status and gender. *J Clin Pharmacol* 2001; 41: 770-8
- Sweeney CT, Fant RV, Fagerström KO, et al. Combination nicotine replacement therapy for smoking cessation: rationale, efficacy and tollerabilità. *CNS Drugs* 2001; 15: 453-67
- Takagi H, Umemoto T. Varenicline: quantifying the risk. *CMAJ* 2011; 183: 1359-66
- Tekle A, al-Khamis KI. Phenytoin-bupropion interaction: effect on plasma phenytoin concentration in the rat. *J Pharm Pharmacol* 1990; 42: 799-801
- Tønnesen P, Carozzi L, Fagerström KO, et al. Smoking cessation in patients with respiratory disease: a high priority, integral component of therapy. *Eur Respir J* 2007; 29: 390-417
- Tonstad S, Tønnesen P, Hajek P, et al; Varenicline Phase 3 Study Group. Effect of maintenance therapy with varenicline on smoking cessation. *JAMA* 2006; 296: 64-71
- Tsai ST, Chi HJ, Cheng HS, et al. A randomized, placebo-controlled trial of varenicline, a selective $\alpha_4\beta_2$ nicotinic acetylcholine receptor partial agonist, as a new therapy for smoking cessation in Asian smokers. *Clin Ther* 2007; 29: 1027-39
- Turpeinen M, Tolonen A, Uusitalo J, et al. Effect of clopidogrel and ticlopidine on cytochrome P450 2B6 activity as measured by bupropion hydroxylation. *Clin Pharmacol Ther* 2005; 77: 553-9
- van Schayck CP, Kaper J, Wagena EJ, et al. The cost-effectiveness of antidepressants for smoking cessation in chronic obstructive pulmonary disease (COPD) patients. *Addiction* 2009; 104: 2110-7
- van Schayck CP, Pinnock H, Ostrem A, et al. IPCRG Consensus statement: tackling the smoking epidemic – practical guidance for primary care. *Prim Care Respir J* 2008; 17: 185-93
- Vetter VL, Elia J, Erickson C, et al. Cardiovascular monitoring of children and adolescents with heart disease receiving medications for attention deficit/hyperactivity disorder: a scientific statement from the American Heart Association Council on Cardiovascular Disease in the Young Congenital Heart Defects Committee and the Council on Cardiovascular Nursing. *Circulation* 2008; 117: 2407-23
- Vogt F, Hall S, Marteau TM. Understanding why smokers do not want to use nicotine dependence medications to stop smoking: qualitative and quantitative studies. *Nicotine Tob Res* 2008; 10: 1405-13
- Wagena EJ, de Vos A, Horwith G, et al. The immunogenicity and safety of a nicotine vaccine in smokers and non smokers: results of a randomized, placebo-controlled phase 1 / 2 trial. *Nicotine Tob Res* 2008; 10: 213-8
- Wagena EJ, Knipschild PG, Huibers MJ, et al. Efficacy of bupropion and nortriptyline for smoking cessation among people at risk for or with chronic obstructive pulmonary disease. *Arch Inter Med* 2005; 165: 2286-92

- Wang C, Xiao D, Chan KP, et al. Varenicline for smoking cessation: a placebo-controlled, randomized study. *Respirology* 2009; 14: 384-92
- Wigger LC, Smets EM, Oort FJ, et al. Adherence to nicotine replacement patch therapy in cardiovascular patients. *Int J Behav Med* 2006; 13: 79-88
- Worrall SP, Almond MK, Dhillon S. Pharmacokinetics of bupropion and its metabolites in haemodialysis patients who smoke. A single dose study. *Nepkron Clin Prucl* 2004; 97: c83-c89

17 The Process of Relapse

Fabio Lugoboni [1]

[1] Department of Internal Medicine, Medical Unit for Addictive Disorders, University of Verona, Policlinico GB Rossi, Verona, Italy

"The son said to him, 'Father, I have sinned against heaven and against you. I am no longer worthy to be called your son."

"But the father said: bring the fatted calf and kill it, and let us eat and make merry; for this my son was dead, and is alive again; he was lost, and is found."

[The Gospel of Luke]

"Giving up smoking is the easiest thing in the world. I know because I've done it thousands of times."

[Mark Twain]

The concept of relapse applies very well to drug addiction, also called chronic relapsing disease, but is not limited to it; the same process can be extended to many areas of behavior and of the medical field. In a broad and shared meaning, relapse is a violation of one or more self-imposed rules determining a defined kind of behavior.

Total abstinence is therefore violated by a single negative "event;" for many schools of thought the pattern is binary: either white or black, in a pattern of:

abstinence > total relapse

For the most rigid educational systems (such as those of several therapeutic communities), the patient is "loaded" at the highest level to deny the possibility of a sporadic use of the substance on which he depended; the regulatory pattern provides for the immediate and unconditional withdrawal at the first offense; in such schemes there is no room for relapse prevention; or better, the complex process of relapse is not analyzed in its explicit form.

But although the violation of the rule represents the main form of relapse, other forms of relapse should be included in the definition.

Let's distinguish then between the first violation of the rule, which we will define as "error," and the subsequent effects in which the patient's behavior can go back closer to the baseline prior to treatment, or relapse with the complete collapse of motivation that we have seen.

The scheme will be:

abstinence > error > total relapse

Relapse is a transition process rather than a failure result; relapse is a series of events that may or may not be followed by a return to baseline levels of "negative" pretreatment behavior: returning to smoking, drinking, etc.

The objective is that, whenever it happens, the error not turn into full relapse.

In this perspective, we must avoid thinking of the individual error as a relapse, seeing it rather as a dangerous crossroads between the right direction and the wrong one.

When the subject maintains complete abstinence, he experiences a feeling of control.

The longer the period of abstinence, the stronger the feeling of self-control through the elimination of discrepancy and increased self-esteem and self-efficacy.

This is of course a good thing: the patient finds not smoking anymore to be "normal." But there is also a negative meaning in all this: the patient gives a relative value to his being abstinent from smoking; now abstinence is **normal**, not special as it was in the early days of abstinence when he felt the satisfaction of the victory. In this normalization of abstinence, dangerous situations are at high risk of occurring.

A high-risk situation is a state which can threaten the self-control of the subject and increase the risk of a potential error.

According to Alan G. Marlatt—who is considered the most eminent scholar of relapse processes—**high-risk situations for relapse are seven**.

The most frequent (approximately 25% of a large sample including smokers, drinkers, and gamblers) is the **alteration of emotional state**, both in a positive and, more frequently, in a negative sense.

The person experiences an emotionally uncomfortable feeling of frustration, anger, anxiety, depression, or boredom that leads to the error; this mood may also be, conversely, strongly positive, characterized by intense euphoria and a sense of omnipotence. In both cases, the result can be dangerous: the person frequently lives through this time as an exceptional situation (both in the positive and in the negative form), outside the normal everyday context, considering it as independent from future consequences.

Marlatt, in his writings, gives the following example:

"It had been raining for a week and I felt sad and bored; I went into the shed and found it completely flooded; then, when I turned on the light, I got an electric shock. Later, after a while, my friend made an estimate of $3,000 for repairs; then I felt that I definitely needed a cigarette, and asked him for one peremptorily."

The second high-risk situation, another frequent cause of relapse, is **interpersonal conflict** in the family, friendship, or business; these are, emotionally, high-involvement situations.

Sometimes, this is experienced by the subject as a form of aggression that is very dangerous for the relationship, and the desire to drink or smoke can become imperious in such cases. It is easy to think that, in reality, when abstinence fails, it was someone else's fault.

Marlatt cites the case of a parent waiting up much of the night for his son, out with his father's car; and when the son is back home, he reprimands him sternly, but the son's answer is an accusation of inconsistency, blaming the father because he's always prying into his business. Then the son leaves the house, slamming the door. At this point, the father feels a strong desire to smoke, despite several months of complete abstinence.

Another important cause of relapse is the situation defined as **social pressure**, a context characterized by a high level of complicity, indifference, or explicit invitation to interrupt the abstinence. The invitation to join in the prohibited behavior may be direct or indirect; what the subject perceives in that context is a very low value attributed to his being abstinent.

The example given by Marlatt, relapse in drinking of an alcoholic after a long-time abstinence, is particularly significant:

> *"I had been involved in a surprise party at my boss's house; I was there rather late, feeling uncomfortable about this, while all of my colleagues were already there and, perfectly at ease, they were all drinking. Then my boss's wife, whom I had never met before, asked me what did I want to drink. I was chilled, and I said, 'J&B on the rocks.'"*

These are the most common high-risk situations, being the cause of relapse in 75% of the cases in a large sample of subjects. Other high-risk situations, however, have to be described.

Self-control verification is a unique and subtle high-risk situation in which the subject, now accustomed to the new behavior, takes up the substance on which he had depended for experimental purposes, out of curiosity rather than frank desire.

> *"One year exactly had passed since I stopped smoking and I did not feel the need at all. I was really in disbelief of the claim, so often heard from friends, that just one cigarette could lead to a relapse. I decided to do an experiment with the only cigarette I had kept as a souvenir."*

Unfortunately, the result is often a repeat of the assumption, leading to a full relapse.

Opportunities are situations in which the subject, quite unexpectedly, encounters the substance. The effect may be, in football terms, that of the "goal on the counterattack."

"After six months of complete abstinence from smoking I found in an old raincoat a package with seven cigarettes. Instinctively, I thought I'd throw them away; but then I thought I would smell them, and then I told myself that they could be a kind of trophy. The following night, walking the dog, I lit one cigarette for curiosity ..."

Illness is another situation predisposing to relapse. The emotion felt by the subject is one of futility about his efforts to change. He stopped smoking, but nevertheless had an angina attack, or fell sick with pneumonia. The subtle thought that everything has been useless, or that smoking is not so dangerous, tends to persuade the subject to relapse.

The **altered state of sobriety**, with its decrease in monitoring capacity, is an important cause of relapse, especially in the consumption of substances. The most frequent medium causing this state is the alcoholic beverage; the subject, even if not frankly abnormal, tends to minimize the risk involved in lighting a cigarette. Even in this situation, a repeat of the error leads, almost invariably, to the reappearance of craving and to complete relapse.

The subtle and implacable mechanism of relapse cannot be fully understood if we don't consider the role played by the **AVE**. When, in one of the seven high-risk situations described, the subject starts taking the drug again after a long or short period of abstinence, an immediate sense of "sin," of having broken a personal vow, is often felt. This sharp sense of transgression causes a powerful and painful reopening of the discrepancy; the pain is strong, intimate, shameful. When the pain is not too strong, the subject puts it to rest by minimizing the accident ("At the end of the day, I did nothing wrong, considering all the cigarettes I'd been smoking before!"); while if the fracture is too far open, the need to use the substance can essentially represent a paradoxical comfort to the inner pain. This state is well described in Antoine de Saint-Exupery's "The Little Prince": in front of the drunk, the Little Prince asks him, "Why are you drinking?" "To forget drinking!" he answers.

The effect of abstinence violation becomes even more deadly when the sudden reopening of the fracture is accompanied by a fall of self-efficacy and by the uncomfortable feeling that everything is useless and relapse is inescapable.

According to Marlatt, the relapse pattern is the following:

exposure to a high-risk situation > inability to cope with the stimulus > error > abstinence violation effect > new failure > reappearance of rewarding effects of the substance > total relapse

If the person maintains a coping response effective in high-risk situations, the probability of relapse decreases because the feeling of self-control increases ("I can also control difficult situations") and the feeling of self-confidence increases as well ("In the future too, I think I can control this situation") [Marlatt, 2008].

Why, sometimes, isn't it possible to cope? The causes can be many:

- The subject no longer recognizes the appropriate value of being abstinent.
- The subject fails to recognize the high-risk situation before it's too late.
- The subject isn't able to ride (or "to surf" in Marlatt's terminology) past the craving moments.
- The reward from the new intake undermines the motivation to resist the temptation.
- The subject falls prey to the AVE [Zgierska, 2009].

The process of relapse must not be considered to be just a temporary distraction at a difficult time; high-risk situations are continually present in everyday life, and external stimuli, such as seeing others smoking, are almost constant.

The process described by Marlatt is more intimate, apparently hidden, and it acts on internal stimuli (much more powerful than the external ones), starting from seemingly insignificant events and negligible choices. The high-risk situation is just the latest stage of a process that began much earlier; as if the subject was put in a situation from which it seems frankly impossible or very difficult to escape.

When the patient tells the unfolding of events, he tends to describe the time of the error with the terms of "fatally," "coincidentally," "to the height of bad luck," "to a tragic fate," etc. Marlatt describes the clinical case of a pathological gambler who relapsed during a company trip. The patient's description to the therapist was of having been dragged, against his will, to Reno (a city in Nevada which is devoted to gambling, on the model of Las Vegas), where he played up to fall heavily.

A more careful analysis of the case showed that the trip had actually been organized by the patient himself, Lake Tahoe being its goal. The fact that nothing was organized for the afternoon, in a place without special attractions, with Reno being so close to the lake, had resulted in someone proposing to extend the trip into town where, fatally, the patient had succumbed to social pressure, starting to play small, leading to a total relapse into pathological gambling. In such cases, the patient seems to project his relapse accurately, despite denying strongly any personal intent in the concatenation of events.

Explaining rationally to the patient what happened can be very difficult because of his strong resistance; recognizing and being able to circumvent that resistance with the techniques of motivational interviewing can be decisive in these cases.

17.1 The Therapist's Role in the Process of Relapse

The role of the therapist is potentially decisive in the recovery from a relapse. It requires a thorough analysis. Very briefly, the context is as follows:

- Our patient relapsed because he did not take the advice and healthy suggestions that we generously provided and this makes him "less attractive."
- The patient tends to minimize ("Come on, Doctor, please do not exaggerate!") or dramatize ("I'm a bad patient, forget me!"), and this makes it more difficult to reverse the error.
- Motivation is greatly suffering, often oscillating between early-contemplation and contemplation; of course, the patient who has relapsed into precontemplation we won't easily see: he usually has little desire to face the issue.
- The external motivations, more fragile and fleeting, tend to prevail over the inner, more intense and enduring: "Honestly, doctor, I came back here just because my wife managed to make me promise."
- In other words, we have a more resistant, more difficult, and less motivated patient ... and we are more skeptical and less helpful.

A nice picture, no doubt about it!

The therapist, beyond the techniques and strategies described above, must synthesize his two roles: a regulatory role and an emotional role. In other words, you might say he needs to use wisely both the stick and the carrot.

We have repeatelly emphasized the fragility, the ambivalence, the irrationality that our recently relapsed patient brings into play—all the unconscious devices he uses to avoid saying simply and clearly: "I realize I have made a series of errors and I promise not to make any more, whatever the cost."

It's clear that if our patient says this, it means that he has become determined, and everything will probably end in the best way; moreover, the errors will serve as a lesson for the future. So everything is okay, but ... this very seldom happens.

Unfortunately, we are very often confronted with a patient swinging from too much self-blame:

"I'm a wimp, I've ruined everything, I have no hope!"

to an irritating minimization of the problem:

"There have been only six or seven cigarettes in a week! You do not know the hell I'm living in at home!"

with the paradoxical tendency to reassure the therapist:

"Don't worry, I just had a heavy week; in four or five days I'll put things right. I'm going to call you soon!"

In this difficult situation the role of the therapist, despite the maximum possible empathy, should be neither that of a tutor, nor of a nanny looking after the patient:

"Call me on your mobile when you want. I'm always available. We can meet at your house. I'm not that hard to find."

nor of an inquisitorial judge:

"You made one of the most serious mistakes of your life and if you don't change your behavior immediately, you're going to suffer very heavy consequences!"

The regulatory role can be summed up in a father's role: a leadership role, demanding full trust in order to achieve the goal, setting the rules of the game firmly and explaining them clearly, but also expecting full respect. The message he wants to convey is "I will be fair but uncompromising. I can give you another chance, but I won't tolerate new mistakes." The role of affection can be summarized in a mother's role: the style is emotional, sympathetic, forgiving, listening, confident; the message she wants to give is: "I'll be your support."

The transition between the two roles must be calculated, ready, careful; and if the patient has a minimizing attitude, you have to point out the discrepancy by focusing on the regulatory role, demonstrating a serious concern about the infringement:

"You have been incautious."

without pushing too hard on the guilt, judging the subject, or making useless generalizations:

"How could you do this after everything we've done so far? You have a tendency not to listen to what you are told!"

This attitude is often more effectively expressed with the nonverbal language of glances or a dismayed shaking of the head, in order to move the patient away from his consolatory defences, the thin crust under which he knows he has committed a serious error.

But just as the careful doctor feels the painful part trying to understand where and how the pain is, ready to retract once its source has been detected, so the regulatory role must give way to emotional support as soon as the discrepancy has been revealed; acute pain can cause resistance, and resistance must be neutralized in the process of relapse.

Facilitating the return to therapy and the return to change is the first priority and the only task. The strategies and techniques to achieve this goal are very important because relapse acts in an emotionally negative way on the therapist also, his patience, his empathy, and, ultimately, his availability. Let's have a look:

- **Normalizing the relapse**. The therapist needs to relieve the strong discrepancy hurting the patient, in order to enhance his self-efficacy, which is very low at this stage. "This is normal for a person starting smoking again after years of quitting; I think you also know many people like me, who did it."
- **Examining carefully the events that led to relapse**. This means shifting the focus of events, reducing the patient's feelings of guilt, and making sure he lives the relapse as an experience not to be repeated, as an opportunity for learning.
- **Demonstrating confidence in the patient's capacity to resume his way to change**. This is a matter of acting directly on the patient's self-efficacy, as we have mentioned several times. Then it is useful to look back ("You were so good the last time, I remember it well, no one was expecting you to stop."), and to look forward assuming the worst ("You feel so hopeless now, but what would happen if you didn't quit smoking?").
- **Trying to avoid by all means making the patient feel guilty**. Guilt, when strong, can easily generate, especially in susceptible individuals, a state of depression which must then be recognized and treated. Often mood assessment is considered a secondary aspect, especially in the field of internal medicine. This is a big mistake because, just when we are asking the patient for a particularly strong commitment, we risk facing his serious apathy.
- **Maintaining a supporting contact**. When it is not possible to take a patient into a path of change, we must at least explain that the door is still open, and we will be happy to talk about it when he decides to try again.

References

- Lugoboni F, Quaglio G, Sarti M, et al. Curing smoking: a priority health objective. *Ann Ital Med Int* 2003; 18: 73-82
- Marlatt GA, Barett K. Relapse prevention. In: Galanter M, Kleber HD (eds). Textbook of Substance Abuse Treatment, 4th Edition. Washington, DC: American Psychiatric Publishing, Inc., 2008
- Zgierska A, Rabago D, Chawla N, et al. Mindfulness meditation for substance use disorders: a systematic review. *Subst Abus* 2009; 30: 266-94

CPSIA information can be obtained
at www.ICGtesting.com
Printed in the USA
LVHW02s1432030518
575858LV00004B/197/P

9 788897 419334